Gentle Healing
with
Homeopathy

Gentle Healing with
with
Homeopathy

*A Practical Primer
to Self-Treatment of
Common Ailments*

INGA-MARIA RICHBERG

Sterling Publishing Co., Inc. New York

Professional Advice by Christine Matthiesen, Physician/Homeopath

Translated by Elisabeth E. Reinersmann
Edited by Lael Kimble, DIHom.

Library of Congress Cataloging-in-Publication Data

Richberg, Inga-Maria.
    [Sanft Heilen mit homöopathie. English]
    Gentle healing with homeopathy: a practical primer to self-treatement
of common ailments / Inga-Maria Richberg; translated by Elisabeth E.
Reinersmann.
        p.   cm.
    Includes index.
    ISBN 0-8069-8112-1
    1. Homeopathy—Popular works. 2. Homeopathy—Materia medica and
therapeutics. I. Title.
RX76. R5413   1997
615.5′32—dc21   97-7715
                                                                                    CIP

10 9 8 7 6 5 4 3 2 1

Published by Sterling Publishing Company, Inc.
387 Park Avenue South, New York, N.Y. 10016
© 1997 by Sterling Publishing Company, Inc.
Original German language edition, *Sanft heilen mit Homöopathie,*
© 1995 by Mosaik Verlag GmbH, Munich / 54321
Distributed in Canada by Sterling Publishing
℅ Canadian Manda Group, One Atlantic Avenue, Suite 105
Toronto, Ontario, Canada M6K 3E7
Distributed in Great Britain and Europe by Cassell PLC
Wellington House, 125 Strand, London WC2R 0BB, England
Distributed in Australia by Capricorn Link (Australia) Pty Ltd.
P.O. Box 6651, Baulkham Hills, Business Centre, NSW 2153, Australia

Sterling ISBN 0-8069-8112-1

For Brita and Christian

TABLE OF CONTENTS

PREFACE

Homeopathy has made a tremendous leap in popularity. As little as 20 years ago, homeopathy existed more or less in the "shadows" as an almost secret science and was vehemently denounced by the established medical profession. But much has changed since then, not the least of which is the birth of the environmental movement and the growing uneasiness with today's five-minute, high-tech medical procedure. But as is so often the case with new trends, the "back-to-nature" movement too overstepped its bounds. Some of the responsibility belongs to the media, who—with sensational reports—made many people believe that so-called "natural" remedies were the answer to all of their ills. It is also not uncommon for people to consider themselves experts in homeopathy just because they have read in a magazine about the successful treatment of an illness with a homeopathic remedy, or had a physician prescribe one for them. All this has done great harm to the reputation of homeopathy, a disservice that has been totally undeserved.

THE DEMANDS OF HOMEOPATHY

Homeopathy is a serious, scientifically proven form of therapy that makes great personal and professional demands on those who are practicing it. Professional qualifications include a well-rounded medical education and training as well as the ability to establish a careful and detailed case history and to participate in an ongoing continuous education. On the personal side, a homeopathic practitioner must always critically and ruthlessly question his own observations and conclusions and be willing to learn from his own daily experiences. In addition, a homeopathic practitioner must always be conscious of the limitations inherent in this treatment modality. Sadly, there are those who do not take their responsibilities as seriously as they should and may, for instance, prescribe medication over the phone without having seen the patient. While this seems very easy, it is nevertheless a serious violation of one of the basic principles of homeopathy.

What is true for the professional homeopathic therapist also holds for the lay person who either wants to treat himself or a family member at home. And here, the limitations are even narrower. Anybody who is thinking of performing such treatments at home must keep this clearly in mind. If this person would be as careless with homeopathic remedies as many are with over-the-counter pain medication—treating according to the motto "More is better"— then it is suggested that they stay away from homeopathy. While a lay person with such an approach will not necessarily cause any real harm, it is still possible to make the symptoms being treated worse or to bring about serious complications.

But those who, on the other hand, are capable of patient and careful observations, are always open to expanding their knowledge, know their own limitations, and are willing to seek professional advice when necessary can do a lot of good, and over time they will develop a deep understanding about the health of the human being. Because homeopathy teaches the person involved to live a healthy lifestyle, and sees to it that family members do likewise, it teaches early intervention when an imbalance in the psychological, mental, or physical equilibrium is detected, and thus is helpful in restoring overall well-being and an ability to enjoy life. And last but not least, it also reduces, to a great degree, the overall financial cost of staying healthy.

Inga-Maria Richberg

Christina Matthiesen

PART I

INTRODUCTION TO HOMEOPATHY

WHAT IS HOMEOPATHY?

Stated in simple terms, homeopathy is a holistic, gentle approach to treating health problems. It is intended to activate a patient's own capacity for self-healing by guiding it into the proper direction and thereby making it possible for the body to overcome the illness on its own. The principles of homeopathy are easy to understand if one takes a look at the history of its development, which is inseparably connected to Samuel Hahnemann. The whole of homeopathy, to this day, is based on his ideas and experiments.

SAMUEL HAHNEMANN, GENIUS AND PHYSICIAN

Born on April 10, 1755, in Meissen, Germany, Samuel Hahnemann was the son of an impoverished artisan. Samuel showed, early on, an extraordinary talent for languages—in the end, speaking eight fluently—and the natural sciences. He studied medicine, and worked for some time as a physician. But he did not enjoy practicing the profession, having become disillusioned by the methods used at the time, some of them quite brutal, such as blood-letting and the use of highly toxic "medications" such as mercury, which seemed to do more harm than good to the patient.

Frustrated, he gave up medicine and began to translate medical and scientific texts and books, something he had already done as a student. Over the years, his work provided him with a immense amount of knowledge that turned out to be a wonderful asset. But he was not only a highly qualified scientist, he also possessed extraordinary intuition.

TRAILBLAZING DISCOVERY

Hahnemann was 35 years old when, in 1790, he translated from English into German a report about the treatment of malaria—or intermittent fever as this illness was called at the time—with China bark. The report claimed that the healing effect of this bark (which came from the China bark tree) was due to the "stomach-strengthening power" of the medication. Hahnemann became curious and spontaneously decided to test the medicine on himself. The result was nothing short of astounding. In every instance, after having taken the medication and within a very short period of time, he would experience for two to three hours symptoms that were similar to those experienced by people with malaria: shivering, cold hands and feet, extreme thirst, intolerable anxiety, dizziness, a feeling of numbness of the whole body, and overwhelming weakness. Or, as Hahnemann described it: China bark—when taken by a healthy person—brought about malaria-like symptoms. This seems to indicate that the benefit of the medication was not its stomach-strengthening effect; there had to be another reason. And here is where Hahnemann's great intuitive sense came to the fore.

"LIKE IS CURED BY LIKE, " THE LAW OF SIMILARS

Hahnemann concluded that it must be the malaria-like symptoms, prompted by the China bark, that stimulated the defense mechanism of the malaria-suffering patient, thereby setting the process of self-healing in motion. From that reasoning followed the conclusion that for a specific illness one only needed to find the proper substance that would produce symptoms similar to that of the illness when it was given to a healthy person. This prompted Hahnemann's formulation of the first principle of this new treatment modality, which he later called homeopathy:

Similia similibus currentur, meaning: let likes be cured by likes

This principle is also called the "Law of Similars," which the term "homeopathy" also defines. Derived from the ancient Greek, homeopathy breaks down into *homoios*, meaning similar, and *pathos*, meaning suffering, or dis-ease. Homeopathy thus translates into similar, or equal, disease.

From the time of his first discovery, Hahnemann dedicated all his energies to the search of finding new homeopathic remedies that corresponded to the Law of Similars, called "Similimum" or "Similia." In the beginning, Dr. Hahnemann looked for different substances and tested them on himself; later, he enlisted the help of family members, students, and colleagues. By his death in 1835 in Paris, Hahnemann, with their support, had scientifically tested close to one hundred substances, declaring each as a Similia for a very specific illnesses. Every reaction and every symptom that these substances activated in healthy people was painstakingly recorded in what he called his Materia Medica. To this day, nothing of the original protocol has been changed. Even the modern Materia Medica of Homeopathy, the collection of the descriptions of homeopathic medications, still follows the protocol established so long ago by Dr. Hahnemann. All in all, more than 2000 substances, all tested according to the

Hahnemann principles, have been found to be Similia and therefore are considered to be homeopathic remedies for very specific symptoms. However, only a small percentage of these substances is used in homeopathy on a day-to-day basis.

HIGHEST PRINCIPLE: ABSOLUTE CERTAINTY

The reason for Hahnemann's insistence on "absolute certainty" when testing substances and then using them for homeopathic remedies can easily be traced back to his earlier experiences with the "highly toxic" medications used in his day, and particularly since he himself was testing such highly toxic substances—arsenic (*Arsenicum album*) was one—for their applicability as Similia. In order to reduce the content of a possibly toxic substance so that it could do no harm, Hahnemann developed an ingenuous system of dilution and succusion (rhythmical shaking) of basic (mother) substances, which not only made the substances less toxic, but also made their healing effect more potent. How much of this technique was based on intuition and how much on observation is difficult to determine with certainty today. As is the case with many people who have made trailblazing discoveries, it is probably a combination of both.

DILUTING

To this day, the technique used for producing homeopathic medications and the procedure for testing new substances for their use as Similia have never changed. The first step is to separate the basic substance. It is taken from plants, minerals, animal products, and sometimes even the products of the human metabolism. This is usually done using alcohol. The result, the so-called homeopathic mother solution, is then—step by step—diluted in a water solution that has a high alcohol content.

For this purpose, Hahnemann established several different scales; the most commonly used today is the centicimal (meaning "to the hundredths") scale, or C scale, where 1 drop of the mother solution is added to 100 drops of the carrier solution. Next, the mixture is shaken in a certain rhythmical fashion in order to, as Hahnemann said, unlock the healing energy of the substance and transfer it to the carrier solution. The result of the first step of dilution is called C1 dilution or, more precisely, a C1 potency. If this solution is again diluted by 1:100, a C2 solution is the result. The dilution process can be continued indefinitely; C1000 or even C50,000 potency are possible and indeed have been used, if only by the very experienced homeopathic physician.

Another scale is the decimal (meaning to the tenth) or D scale, where the mother solution and all additional potencies are diluted each at a ratio of 1:10. In addition, homeopathy deals with Q and LM ratios that have, however, no relevance for the lay person.

POTENTIZATION

"Potentization" of a remedy, by serial dilution and rhythmical shaking, is somewhat confusing to the lay person. How Hahnemann arrived at this technique, as already stated, is not known with certainty. But one thing is certain: behind the idea of potentization is a thought that is as simple as it is brilliant.

The apparent paradox of homeopathic remedies can be reduced to a short formula: the more diluted a solution, the more potent it is. This principle has given rise to the term "potentization." Even when the final solution contains no identifiable trace of the medication, if it still elicits the symptoms of a specific illness when administered to a healthy person, it is the correct Similia to be used, and it will effect sustained healing in the sick person. Responsible for this phenomenon, Hahnemann thought, was the healing energy of the mother solution, which, with increasing dilution, was obviously transferred unadulterated to the carrier solution. One could also view this phenomenon as a kind of energy fingerprint of the mother tincture in the carrier solution: the smaller the amount of disruptive matter, the more pure the imprint of the healing energy.

That homeopathic remedies are effective—even if no molecules of the mother solution are present (in the case of C-solution this happens at about C9, and in D-solutions from D30 on)—is the most difficult principle for the medical profession to understand, and it is not surprising that homeopathy is dismissed by most with the objection, "There is nothing there; therefore, it cannot work!" This is one of the most constantly repeated arguments against homeopathic remedies. But something obviously *is* present in these highly diluted solutions. It's just that we are not yet able to prove it with the measuring techniques available today. Maybe someday physics will be able to. For instance, let's look at a past assumption: for the longest time, people simply smiled dismissively when it was suggested that plants are surrounded by an aura of electrical waves. But, lo and behold, the invention of Kirilian photography made it possible to prove to the skeptics that they were wrong. And did we not believe at one time that the Earth was flat?

THE BASIC PRINCIPLES OF HOMEOPATHIC TREATMENT

This central premise of homeopathic treatment was also developed by Dr. Hahnemann: "Treat the person, not the illness."

Homeopathy starts with the premise that a person is not *getting* sick but that he or she *is* sick, which means that the individual's physical, mental, and psychological balance has been disturbed. For a homeopathic physician, a person's symptoms are a healthy sign that the body's self-healing power is attempting to reestablish its balance. It is the function of homeopathic treatment to support this process. What kind of support is needed is shown by the person's symptoms, which are the result of the body's attempt to heal itself.

Since the homeopath treats the whole person and not merely the illness, there is less interest in "naming" an illness than in the individual symptoms that are indicative of a disease. The deciding factor is that the medication given to the sick person is appropriate for the whole person. No medication is prescribed for an illness. Accordingly, the emphasis is on a very thorough and detailed inquiry of each individual complaint. This is the only way in which the homeopath is able to determine which remedy is appropriate in any given situation. How this is done is discussed in general terms in the following pages. This very basic principle is also relevant when homeopathic remedies are used by the lay person in the home.

THE HOMEOPATHIC CASE HISTORY

The recording of the complaints, or anamnesis, is usually a two-part process. First, the patient is asked to accurately explain the nature of the complaint bringing him or her to the office. Then, the homeopath tries to determine if any other symptoms are present that would make the choice of medication easier. During this phase, the homeopath literally checks out the patient's body from the head down to the toes, includes in his inquiry the patient's mental and psychological state, and considers the experiences and situations in the patient's life, as well as any prior important events.

Particularly important in deciding which medication is appropriate is the so-called modality, where the patient is asked if the complaints are better or worse under certain circumstances. The four modalities generally considered are: rest, motion, cold, or warmth. These are further modified and expanded on—for instance, movement in fresh air, etc.

Choosing the Proper Medication

After the case history has been conducted—which in the case of chronic complaints may take two hours or several office appointments—the homeopath will choose the proper Similia: the remedy that matches the characteristics of the symptoms. Sometimes the choice is obvious, and sometimes several different remedies are needed; in some cases, the patient needs none at all. In any case, the homeopath must compare scrupulously the characteristics of the symptoms—with the help of the Materia Medica—against those of the medications that he is considering. Only when both coincide, whereby not all symptoms listed need to be present in the patient, may a person prescribe a particular medication. This explains why a homeopathic practitioner will not always prescribe a medication but, instead, may suggest a waiting and observation period during which the nature of the symptoms might become clearer.

Of course, homeopathy, too, has so-called proven indicators, distinct characteristics of a complaint or symptom, that tell the experienced practitioner which specific remedy is most effective. For instance, in the case of a stabbing pain in the throat that is accompanied by highly inflamed and swollen tissue, the *Apis mellifica* remedy is always the proper medication to use. But even when those reliable indicators are present, the homeopath must always check his choice to assure himself that those symptoms have indicated what indeed is called for in a particular situation.

Only One Remedy at a Time

Another important and central principle of traditional homeopathy, according to Dr. Samuel Hahnemann, states: *Always use only one remedy at a time.*

Behind this principle is the experience that, if more than one remedy has been used, it is impossible to determine which medication has been responsible for the success. In addition, a wrong remedy could itself cause symptoms that can easily misrepresent the original complaints and in turn make the treatment either more difficult or even altogether impossible. It is also possible that no improvement has taken place, and that the medication was the right one but the potency was incorrect. If a patient has been given more than one medication, it is impossible to determine which was the proper one or if only the potency was wrong.

THE CHOICE OF POTENCY

After the proper medication has been chosen, the practitioner must then decide on the specific potency; however, this subject is approached differently by different homeopaths. Some prefer the lower potency of the D-scale (up to D12), while others like to work with the higher potency of the C-scale (up to C30), and still others prefer those with the highest potency of the Q-scale. The average homeopath, however, does not use just one specific potency but rather will make decisions according to the situation of each individual patient. While much depends on the personal experience and intuition of the practitioner, homeopathy has three general guidelines that are the result of long-standing practical experience:

▫ Low-potency remedies (up to D12) affect mainly the body. From D12 upward, mental/psychological effects are more prominent.
▫ Higher-potency medications usually work faster, go deeper, and last longer—sometimes for weeks or even months longer—than those with a lower potency. Remedies that have higher potencies therefore belong in the hands of the experienced physician and homeopath.
▫ Patients with a strong constitution and a strong defense mechanism—this usually includes children—will activate their body's self-healing ability with lower-potency remedies. Patients who are weaker, on the other hand, usually need higher-potency medication because their self-healing mechanism needs stronger and more effective stimulation.

WHEN TO TAKE MEDICATION

How often a remedy is taken also depends on each individual situation and the specific potency chosen. But here too the homeopath follows two very basic rules, which, again, are based on long-standing experience:

- Low-potency medications are taken more often, because their effects diminish faster. Higher-potency remedies are usually taken only once.
- Medication is discontinued as soon as improvements of the complaints have set in.

Lay people are usually surprised when they hear the second rule, because it is so fundamentally different from conventional medical therapy. But it is easily explained: a distinct improvement of a complaint is an indication that the body's own healing mechanism has been stimulated, and the remedy has done its job. Only if the healing process stagnates—which causes the old complaints to return—or if totally new symptoms appear is it necessary to continue the medication or to choose a new one. If such is the case, the choice of the new remedy again must be checked against the characteristics of the symptoms described in the Materia Medica. It is not unusual that a patient's physical, psychological, and mental imbalance takes different forms in the course of the healing process.

INITIALLY, SYMPTOMS WORSEN

To ascertain if a prescribed medication is really the right one is usually determined by observing the so-called "initial worsening of the symptoms." This means that, after taking the medication, the patient's complaints will initially get worse and then begin to improve slowly. This phenomenon is also easy to explain: homeopathic remedies cause very specific symptoms in a healthy person, a response that, of course, also holds true for a sick person. If, therefore, the symptoms worsen initially, it means that the sick person is responding to the remedy in the same way that a healthy person would, given the stronger dose. In other words, the remedy is right on the mark.

How quickly can one expect the initial complaints to worsen? That also depends on the potency of the prescribed remedy: with a very low potency the complaints will get worse rather quickly, usually within a few hours. But improvement is also very dramatic. If the potency of the remedy is higher, it goes much deeper, and therefore takes somewhat longer until the remedy begins to take effect. The time can be anywhere from one day to even three to four weeks. Of course, it all depends on the complaints, whether they are acute or chronic.

The Healing Process

After the initial worsening of the symptoms, the healing process—following the so-called Hering Law (named after Konstantin Hering, the discoverer of this process)—begins. Hering observed that the physical symptoms begin to heal only after the emotional/psychological complaints have improved. Additional observations consistently show that the healing process follows the following pattern:

- from top to bottom
- from inside out
- from the present to the past

This pattern can most easily be observed in chronic illnesses that have existed for several weeks or months. But in acute illnesses, too, even a lay person with a trained eye can observe this pattern, even if it is not expressed quite as strongly. This is particularly the case when the complaints involve only one organ.

Let's take as an example the case where a person has a severe cold with an intense cough. Before the physical symptoms begin to improve, the patient usually starts to "feel" better. This can be observed most easily in children because—in general—they don't have their emotions as well under control as adults. Once they feel emotionally better and more accepting of the illness, the nose begins to be less stuffed up and secretion begins to flow. The pain in the throat lessens, coughing is less painful, and expectoration becomes easier. The joints ache less, the circulatory system gets back to normal, appetite returns, and the digestive system gets going again. The patient becomes stronger by the day until all is well again.

In acute illnesses as well, it is not all that unusual that the healing process suddenly stops and can only be set in motion again by giving the patient another homeopathic remedy—or a repeat dosage of the original. But here, too, the healing process always follows the Hering Law until healing is complete.

What Can Homeopathy Do?

In general, homeopathy is a highly effective method of treatment even for severely acute as well as chronic diseases. It can even intervene successfully in life-threatening situations. The prerequisite, however, is that the treatments are done by an experienced, professional homeopath who has also been trained and has experience in conventional therapies. In Germany, only physicians are allowed to perform homeopathic treatment. The exception may be a health practitioner who has been thoroughly educated, has long years of practical experience to his credit, and works in close cooperation with a physician. But in spite of the fact that homeopathy is highly effective, it is, like all other forms of therapies, not all-powerful.

LIMITATIONS OF HOMEOPATHY

Stated in simple terms, homeopathy is not useful where the ability of a patient's own capacity for healing is too weak or altogether absent. This is particularly true where one or several organs are severely affected. Other limitations are acute medical emergencies (serious injuries due to accidents) or severe loss of blood. Also, acute breakdown of the circulatory system (heart attack, stroke, lung aneurysm), life-threatening complications during birth, and severe psychiatric illnesses and psychotic disorders all need the help and attention of conventional medicine. It is not that homeopathy could not in general influence the healing process, even in such cases, effectively. It is rather the lack of appropriately trained physicians, especially in hospitals, that accounts for much of homeopathy's disuse.

SELF-TREATMENT WITH HOMEOPATHY

Homeopathy used by the lay person at home is only recommended for light to minor acute complaints, many of which are discussed in this book. Chronic illnesses should always be treated by a professional homeopath. A chronic illness, by definition, is one where complaints have usually been allowed to worsen over many years, and therefore the characteristics of the symptoms have changed several times. To uncover and remove the various layers of symptoms and achieve permanent healing requires not only a tremendous amount of knowledge and experience but also, as we have stated previously, the intuition that only an experienced professional homeopath has acquired. Any extraneous or improper medication can alter or worsen the character of a chronic illness to the point where healing not only becomes very cumbersome but also, under the worst-case scenario, healing may become impossible altogether.

NINE BASIC PRINCIPLES FOR SELF-TREATMENT IN HOMEOPATHY

If you want to treat yourself, or a member of your family, you must proceed, in principle, the same way a professional homeopath would; however, you must strictly adhere to the following nine basic rules:

1. Only treat everyday, acute complaints and illnesses.
2. If you have experienced a great emotional crisis recently, let a professional homeopath treat you and the members of your family.
3. Never, on your own, discontinue the conventional medication prescribed by your physician and take homeopathic remedies instead. You could create a life-threatening situation.
4. Do not treat acute symptoms that develop in the course of treating chronic problems yourself. Always check with your homeopath.
5. Be particularly careful when treating children. Illnesses in children often progress very rapidly. Infants and small children should only be treated when they are under the observation of a physician, because seemingly harmless illnesses can very quickly develop complications; some situations can even become life-threatening.
6. Check the characteristics of the symptoms that you have identified against those listed for a specific medication, paying special attention to the mental/emotional symptoms and circumstances (modalities). If you can't decide what to do, ask a professional homeopath for advice.
7. Always use only one medication at time.
8. If the patient's situation worsens or if high fever sets in, get in touch with your physician immediately.
9. When in doubt, always ask for medical advice, and do so more often rather than not often enough.

ADVICE FOR THE FIRST-TIME USER

If you have decided to give homeopathy a try, never attempt to treat an illness that involves fever. Rather, let your first experience be a really simple malady, and always treat yourself first. Well suited for first-time treatments, for example, are small injuries (cuts and insect bites, but not if a person has allergies!), scratches, or small burns of the skin that under normal circumstances you wouldn't even treat with remedies from your medicine cabinet or cover with a bandage. While a lay person can't do much harm with small complaints, much experience can be gained firsthand about how homeopathy works. Among other things, you will become acquainted with the special language used to describe symptoms that many a lay person finds is rather "flowery." For example, it makes a great deal of difference when choosing the appropriate remedy if the insect bite causes a "burning," "itching," or "biting" sensation, or if the pain gets better when exposed to cold or warmth.

Only after you have practiced on small complaints for a while, and have acquired a good feel for homeopathic remedies, should you go on to more difficult cases like colds that include a runny nose, cough, and aching joints.

HOW TO USE THIS BOOK

This book is based on proven indicators used in homeopathy for a long time. Therefore it is organized according to the main complaints. Let's take, once more, a cold as an example. Depending on how a cold is manifesting itself, either with a runny nose or more in the form of a sore throat and cough, look for the respective term—for instance, Colds, in the chapter Respiratory Problems, Part II—and use the remedy according to the character of the symptoms. Next, compare the character of the complaints you have identified with those listed in the Materia Medica, Part III*. Only when both coincide—though the illness does not need to display all of the symptoms listed—have you found the proper remedy. If not, start from the beginning, paying special attention to the correct description of the symptoms and the modalities under which they either get worse or better.

IMPORTANT: Some illnesses and health problems manifest themselves through different symptoms and do not necessarily involve a certain organ or specific part of the body. This is particularly true for emotional and nervous complaints. For instance, emotional stress may cause stomach problems that appear as intestinal distress. But stress may also cause nervous restlessness, irritation, anxiety, sleeplessness, headaches, and problems during menstruation. In such situations, look under the emotional/psychological term that may also be listed in other chapters.

*The Materia Medica lists those remedies most often used for homeopathic self-treatment. Other, proven remedies produce only one or two symptoms and, therefore, are used less often. These have not been mentioned because of space restrictions. When in doubt, ask your homeopath for advice.

POTENCY, DOSAGE, AND SCHEDULE

How much, when, and how often a specific medication is taken depends on its potency. Particularly useful for home treatment are two potencies: D6 and D12. If no specific potencies are listed, you may freely choose which one you want to use. The following is recommended:

◻ The beginner without experience, who intends to treat another person or himself homeopathically, should use D6 potency.
◻ Those with experience may choose the D12 potency.
◻ If in doubt, ask your homeopath what the proper potency should be in any given situation.

Homeopathic remedies are offered in four different forms; however, not every medication is available in all four forms. The main reason for this, more than anything else, is a function of the manufacturing process. The four different forms are drops (dilutions), globuli, tablets, and powder (used for trituration). The last three of these forms consist of lactose to which a specific potency has been added. In general, all four forms are taken orally. In addition, some remedies come in vials and are injected; of course, this type is not used for home treatment.

◻ The standard dosage: 5 drops, 5 globuli, 1 tablet, or 1 pinch of powder for trituration.

Which one of the four different types you chose is a matter of preference. Experience has shown that most people prefer to take homeopathic remedies in the form of drops or globuli; the latter work particularly well for children because they are free of alcohol, are easy to take, taste good, and are very small. In the case of highly acute complaints, some remedies (specifically marked in Part II) are used in the following manner: drops, globuli, tablets, or powder are dissolved in half a glass of water, which is then sipped or taken by the spoonful until the patient gets better. IMPORTANT: Do not use a metal spoon, only those made of plastic or porcelain.

◻ Medicine is taken either 2 hours before or 1 hour after a meal. Do not swallow the medication with water or similar liquids; rather, allow it to dissolve in the mouth or, better yet, under the tongue.

Since low-potency medication is effective for a shorter time than is high-potency, the following schedule, unless stated otherwise, is recommended for standard dosage:

D6 Potency

◻ Take every hour for the first 6 hours; if there is improvement, reduce to three times a day until improvement stabilizes; then, discontinue medication.
◻ If no improvement is noticed after 6 hours, choose another remedy; if there is still no improvement, see your physician.

D12 Potency

◻ In the beginning, 3 times daily. If improvement sets in after one day, reduce to once a day until improvement is stabilized; then discontinue medication.
◻ In case of severe complaints, every 30–60 minutes until improvement sets in; however, use no more than 5 standard dosages.
◻ If there is no improvement after one day of treatment, switch to another remedy; if this too does not bring improvement, see your physician.

IMPORTANT: Homeopathic remedies can be strongly affected or even totally negated by certain substances. Among these are peppermint, camphor, eucalyptus, menthol, as well as coffee and cola drinks. The fragrance of intensive perfumes can also interfere with the healing energies of a medication. Avoid all of the above while treating complaints with homeopathic remedies. Also, if possible, use a peppermint-free toothpaste. Black tea, unless it is consumed in huge amounts, is permissible. Substituting fruit teas for herbal teas with distinct medicinal properties may be helpful in proper treatment.

◻ If by chance more globuli or tablets have come out of the bottle than you intended, do not return them; rather, throw them away.

A Special Case: Constitutional Remedies

Generally speaking, treatment with constitutional remedies should be left to a professional homeopath because it requires a very involved anamnesis. But it has happened during self-treatment, that a patient reacts to the same medication over and over again, even though expressed complaints vary. Homeopathy considers this to be a constitutional problem that requires treatment with constitutional remedies. For instance, children often present complaints and are in emotional situations that have *Pulsatilla*, *Sulfur*, or *Lycopodium* characteristics. A homeopath will then talk about the child as having a *Pulsatilla*, *Sulfur*, or *Lycopodium* personality. If you are confronted with such a portrait, even if you are very sure of your conclusion, leave constitutional therapy to an experienced homeopath, because such therapy has very far-reaching effects and belongs to the same category as chronic diseases, requiring the utmost care. Also, most homeopaths who do constitutional therapy use high- to extremely high-potency remedies, and they also may use a complicated schedule whereby the potency of the remedy is increased steadily over the course of the treatment. The experience that is necessary to implement such a therapy goes far beyond the capabilities of the lay person.

PART II

TREATING EVERYDAY COMPLAINTS AND ILLNESSES AT HOME WITH HOMEOPATHIC REMEDIES

CHAPTER 1

EMOTIONAL AND NERVOUS COMPLAINTS

BASIC INFORMATION

Emotional and nervous complaints, like increased irritability, lack of concentration, and anxiety, are symptoms that show that energy reserves are at a very low point and are out of balance. The reason can be any number of traumatic events, such as the death of a significant person, separation from or the loss a job because of mental fatigue or overwork, running all the way to a deeply rooted doubt about the values and goals in one's life. Also, suppressed, painful, or uncomfortable experiences in the past can reemerge years later in an seemingly unrelated context. But psychological imbalance does not always manifest itself in emotional/mental complaints; it also shows up in the form of physical complaints. In medicine these are called psychosomatic illnesses. They may affect the heart, the respiratory system, digestion, as well as the skin. All these problems are created through a very complex interaction of the central and vegetative nervous system and the influence of the hormones. However, some elements of this interactive process have yet to be discovered.

When treating a person homeopathically, the precise biochemical mechanism of emotional and psychosomatic symptoms is not all that important. Since the focus is on the whole person, homeopathy is interested in the patient's overall condition.

Each psychological crisis, no matter how uncomfortable its accompanying symptoms may be, has a very distinct and personal message for the individual. The message, no matter how obscure, usually points to what a person must do for himself in order to get better. Our action-oriented world, however, leaves little room for reflection, but forces body, soul, and spirit more and more often to "pull the emergency break" just to get us to slow down. This also explains why, during a personal crisis, we sometimes lose our otherwise perfectly sufficient mental capacities and are unable to concentrate on the daily tasks at hand. Paying attention to our innermost needs, rather than concentrating on external considerations, is what we are asked to do. A small crisis that, under normal circumstances, we can handle easily by ourselves can grow larger if we don't pay attention. Homeopathic remedies can aid us in regaining our inner balance. In the event of a more serious crisis—one that seems to dominate our every day life and lingers on—it is better to seek advice from your physician or homeopath. This also applies to smaller complaints if they are connected to a profound and personally serious crisis or if—in spite of self-treatment—no improvement is noticeable after one week.

When Do You Need to See a Physician

The following is a list of complaints that require you to see a physician (or go to an emergency room):

- if emotional or nervous complaints set in while suffering from a serious, acute illness, such as an infection accompanied by high fever or severe pain
- when undergoing hormonal changes, as during puberty and pregnancy, after a birth, while nursing, during menopause; also when taking home-opathic remedies (including birth-control pills)
- in cases of nervous/emotional problems during chronic illnesses, including metabolic diseases like diabetes
- in cases of severe depression
- in cases of confusion and/or disorientation
- in cases of attacks of severe anxiety
- when losing touch with reality, when experiencing hallucinations and/or delusions
- in cases of aggression
- in cases of having thoughts of suicide

Dosage and Potency

In cases of acute problems, such as anxiety attacks, a standard dosage of a D12 remedy should be taken every 30 minutes until improvement sets in. But this process should not continue for more than two hours; after five standard doses, the remedy should be taken less frequently. After acute treatment, a standard dose of D12 should be taken once a day until improvement is noticeable.

IRRITABILITY

Usually the early sign of strain and overwork, irritability can also be due to a fear of failure or a crisis in a relationship. Family problems can play a major role. This symptom is often coupled with sadness, fear, nervous restlessness, mood swings, and insomnia. Dosage: page 31.

KEY SYMPTOMS	REMEDY
Very irritable, raging, angry; sitting still, withdrawn, sad and silent. Worry about the future. *Worse:* in the morning, cold, when comforted, noise *Better:* at rest, warmth, sleep	**Acidum hydrochloricum**
Irritable, impatient; reserved, won't talk about problems; angry if not left alone. Worry about the future, overwhelmed. *Worse:* in the morning, by motion *Better:* at rest, fresh air	**Bryonia**
Highly irritated, restless, temper tantrums, overly sensitive, dissatisfied; doesn't know what he/she wants; exaggerated reaction to every demand, anger. *Worse:* in the evening, during the night, when touched, when angry, coffee *Better:* when left/being alone, driving a car	**Chamomilla**
Quickly angered, offended, impatient, overwrought by worry, rage, sees only the worst, everything "affects" the stomach. *Worse:* when excited, talking *Better:* warmth, rest/quiet, coffee	**Colocynthis**

KEY SYMPTOMS	REMEDY
Extreme temper tantrums, doesn't want to be talked to, brooding about moral dilemma, worries. Fears contracting an incurable disease. Makes mistakes when writing, reading, talking. *Worse:* when comforted *Better:* in fresh air	**Lilium tigrinum**
Irritable, becomes choleric because of fear of failure, particularly when confronted with anything new; pretends to be strong, dominant, controlling, angry; "sharp tongued." *Worse:* in the morning, between 4 and 8 P.M., and when clothing is too tight *Better:* when moving, in fresh air	**Lycopodium**
Extreme rage due to mental fatigue/over-stimulation of the senses. Impatient, ambitious, pedantic, hypochondriacal; often involves the misuse of medication and stimulants. Particularly for men. *Worse:* worries at work, confrontations, cold *Better:* after a short nap, resting, in the evening	**Nux vomica**
Rage, fighting with others due to total exhaustion, verbally abusive. Particularly for working women and mothers. *Worse:* cold; stuffy air *Better:* sleep, moving outside	**Sepia**
Episodes of extreme rage after having suppressed anger for a long time, shaking when extremely excited, extremely sensitive to what others say about them, suffer much from lack of assertion. *Worse:* when excited, eating, drinking *Better:* during the night, rest, warmth, walking, fresh air	**Staphysagria**

SADNESS AND DEPRESSION

If there is severe depression and extreme hopelessness as well as an increasing use of alcohol and medication, seek advice from your physician and an experienced homeopath immediately. Dosage: page 31.

KEY SYMPTOMS	REMEDY
Internal numbness, apathetic, sad, hopeless. Does not want to be spoken to. Also for lovesickness, homesickness, and during puberty. *Worse:* exertion *Better:* quiet, warmth, when shown sympathy	**Acidum phosphoricum**
Everything is closing in, unsure, shy, anxious, blocked, jittery, insomnia. After mental and emotional exhaustion. *Worse:* music, when given sympathy *Better:* distracted, motion outdoors	**Ambra grisea**
Sudden breakdown, with utter feeling of worthlessness. Loner; can't handle criticism. Particularly intense after failure/mistakes at work. *Worse:* in cold weather, when getting cold *Better:* motion, music	**Aurum metallicum**
Sad, reflective, desire to alone, weak. Anxiety at night; feels abandoned. *Worse:* eating, cold *Better:* warmth	**Carbo animalis**
Melancholy, feels sorry for self, anxious, cries easily; particularly with long-lasting grief, and with increasing age. *Worse:* in the morning *Better:* damp weather, when comforted	**Causticum**

KEY SYMPTOMS	REMEDY
Absent, talks little, moody, easily offended, upset; basically gentle and shy; profound sadness, cannot bear injustice or contradiction; slow to comprehend. *Worse:* noise, driving *Better:* after short nap	**Cocculus**
Spontaneous spells of crying and rage; otherwise introvert, very emotional, romantic. Highly sensitive to insignificant rejections. *Worse:* stimulation, when given sympathy *Better:* sighing, while eating	**Ignatia**
Anxious sadness after sleep; otherwise painful inner restlessness, incessant talk, suspicious, jealous. Cannot bear anything tight anywhere. Particularly for people in menopause and for lovesickness. *Worse:* after sleep, closing eyes *Better:* warm applications	**Lachesis**
Profound sadness, constantly close to tears, has moral dilemmas; fears incurable disease. Making mistakes when reading, writing, and speaking. *Worse:* warmth, touch *Better:* in fresh air	**Lilium tigrinum**
Music causes depression; person is restless, whiny, needs to lie down, shy around people; feels a void between self and others. *Worse:* when weather changes, thunderstorms, in the morning *Better:* by moving	**Natrum carbonicum**

KEY SYMPTOMS	REMEDY
Introverted, sad, serious, holds grudges; constantly thinks about old hurts, can't stand to be comforted, wants to be alone and then starts to cry. *Worse:* in the morning	**Natrum chloratum**
Gentle, good-natured, forgiving, timid, sad, silent grief; surrenders to fate; worries about the future. *Worse:* rest, warmth of any kind *Better:* when given sympathy	**Pulsatilla**
Very sad and exhausted, cries easily; feels abandoned and helpless; unable to care for family after overexertion. Particularly for working women and mothers. *Worse:* cold, stuffy air *Better:* sleep, moving outside	**Sepia**

FEAR

Fear is an essential emotion because it alerts us to possible danger ahead. Fear becomes a problem only when it is out of proportion to a given event. Unreasonable fears, however, are a very distinctive signal, alerting us to the fact that our emotions are out of balance. If everyday activities are severely hampered by fear and the following remedies do not bring relief within 3 days, seek advice from your physician or homeopath. See Stage Fright and Panic Attacks. Dosage: page 31.

KEY SYMPTOMS	REMEDY
Extreme fear with foreboding, panic attacks with fear of death, nightmares, pounding pulse, dizziness, difficulty breathing; feelings of apprehension, hot flashes, red face. Often after emotional shock. *Worse:* nights, around midnight, from hearing music	**Aconitum**

KEY SYMPTOMS	REMEDY

Growing anxiety after overwork; endures for
a long time, then suddenly collapses; fear of
death. Especially for pedantic, and performance-
oriented people.
Worse: when alone, night, after midnight
Better: warmth, cold drinks

Arsenicum album

Fear of infectious diseases, of bad luck;
is confused, forgetful, afraid to lose
his mind, stubborn.
Worse: at night, after mental exertion
Better: quiet, warmth, when feeling secure

Calcarea carbonica

Nervous, anxious, tired, frightened, in
constant fear; can't be in a dark room; totally
exhausted, withdrawn.
Worse: in the morning, cold
Better: in the afternoon, warmth

Kali carbonicum

Fear of failure, especially when doing new things.
Pretends to be strong; haughty; has self-doubt
but is very intelligent, a quick learner.
Worse: in the afternoon, evening, warmth
Better: in fresh air, motion

Lycopodium

Fear with deep depression; often after
excessive worry; very serious; is afraid
to make a fool of himself; anxious in
small spaces; in a crowd, a tendency to faint.
Worse: before noon, for heat, sun, when given
sympathy
Better: when outdoors

Natrum chloratum

Overly sensitive to external influences; takes
everything to heart; extremely afraid of being
alone; fear of thunderstorms, also fear of the
future, sickness, darkness, burglary, and misfortune.
Worse: from things influencing the senses,

Phosphorus

KEY SYMPTOMS	REMEDY

during twilight, at change in weather
Better: getting attention, rest, and sleep

General anxiety; fear of being alone, darkness,   **Pulsatilla**
ghosts; also fear of future; people who are
clinging, are shy, and moody; also for children.
Worse: warmth in any form
Better: outdoors, fresh air, motion

Fear of being overworked; everything is   **Sepia**
too much; tries to avoid others, including
family, but does not want to be alone.
Frequently for working women and mothers.
Worse: in the evening
Better: motion

Incapacitating fear of failure and of   **Silicea**
responsibilities; easily discouraged; makes
himself small; can't think; whiny, needs
protection; common in children.
Worse: exertion, sensory impressions
Better: warmth, fresh air

STAGE FRIGHT AND TEST ANXIETY

The main reason for stage fright and a fear of taking tests is a lack of self-confidence. If the fear is so great that you can't even show up for a test, it is important to seek advice from an experienced homeopath. Dosage: page 31.

KEY SYMPTOMS	REMEDY
Lack of concentration and poor memory; aversion to work; delays working for tests; uncontrollable urge to run away; ravenous appetite.	**Anacardium**
Nervous, overstressed; must do everything in a hurry; always expecting the worst; studying/working up to the last minute; ravenous appetite for sweets; nervous; stomach cramps; diarrhea, increased pulse, jitters.	**Argentum nitricum**
Somewhat exhausted, timid, shy, fearful; increasing restlessness, constant urge to urinate; diarrhea, headaches, heart problems, signs of numbness, jitters; mental block during test, feels paralyzed, can't speak. Affects actors, singers, speakers.	**Gelsemium**
Fear of failure; can't think; easily discouraged, thinks he is small	**Silicea**

SIMPLE PHOBIAS

Phobias are considered fears that are exaggerated and unreasonable in light of the event. Simple phobias are geared towards places, objects, and animals. If your everyday activities are seriously affected by such phobias, seek advice form a physician or homeopath. Dosage: page 31.

KEY SYMPTOMS	REMEDY
Fear of height, small spaces, standing in, crowds, and flying. Sudden impulse to jump off a bridge or balcony but pulling back at the last moment. Nervous, overly excited, overworked; always expecting the worst. *Better:* fresh air, cold	**Argentum nitricum**
Phobic fear of large animals, particularly horses and dogs.	**Causticum**
Phobic fear of: thunderstorms, illness, accidents, being alone, darkness. Highly sensitive toward all external influences. *Worse:* sensory impressions, twilight, change in the weather *Better:* when shown care; rest; sleep	**Phosphorus**
Phobic fear of being alone in the evening and in the dark; of the opposite sex. People who are dependent, shy, but moody. Also children who are unable to go to sleep without a light. *Worse:* warmth in any form *Better:* outdoors, fresh air, motion	**Pulsatilla**
Phobic fear of needles; is looking for them and counting them.	**Silicea**
Phobic fear of pointed objects: needles and knives.	**Spigelia**

KEY SYMPTOMS	REMEDY
Phobic fear of small spaces/rooms and public transportation, particularly a fear of being on trains.	**Succinum**

PANIC ATTACKS AND AGORAPHOBIA

Panic attacks are severe, sudden attacks of fear, including fear of death, for which there seem to be no identifiable reasons. They seem to come out of the blue. They often happen in overly stressful situations: overwork combined with lack of sleep or after emotional exhaustion. One could arise, for instance, because of the death of a loved one or separation from a partner. Those who suffer from repeated panic attacks, over months or even years, and can leave the house only with the greatest of effort (agoraphobia), should seek help from a physician or psychologist immediately. Behavioral therapy has been found to be particularly effective. Here, too, homeopathic remedies can greatly support the healing process. But discuss with your physician or therapist if you want to use homeopathic remedies. Dosage: page 31.

KEY SYMPTOMS	REMEDY
Extreme panic with fear of death; racing pulse, dizziness; difficulty breathing; fullf of apprehension; hot flashes; flushed face. *Worse:* in enclosed spaces, in public places *Better:* at home, in company of trusted person	**Aconitum**
Feeling anxious, particularly when standing in line; crowds; enclosed spaces; always in a hurry; nervous; agitated, feeling of doom; can't handle warmth; ravenous appetite for sweets; nervous stomach cramps; diarrhea; pounding heart; jittery. *Worse:* after a meal *Better:* fresh air, cold, lying down on left side	**Argentum nitricum**

KEY SYMPTOMS	REMEDY

Agoraphobia; feels dead tired; often after exhaustion; after physical overwork and shock; headache with dizziness; stabbing pain in the chest; restlessness; won't talk about what is wrong; wants to be alone.
Worse: touch, motion, rest, wine, damp cold
Better: lying down with the head lower than the feet on a soft surface

Arnica

Acute attack of fear, often with increasing intensity up to fear of death; pounding heart; breathing difficulty, often with cramps in the breathing passage; feeling of apprehension; restlessness; cold sweats; jittery; stomach pain; diarrhea. Particularly for pedantic people and those fixated on performance.
Worse: with exertion, at night, after midnight, when alone
Better: familiar environment and persons

Arsenicum album

Attacks of fear after mental overwork and over-stimulation of the senses; ambitious; choleric; pedantic; hypochrondriacal; misuses of medication and stimulants.
Worse: worries at work, financial worries, light, noise, smells, cold, outdoors
Better: short nap, rest, in the evening

Nux vomica

RESTLESSNESS

Restlessness is often accompanied by other complaints, like exhaustion, fearfulness, lack of concentration, irritability, and insomnia. For that reason, also look up those terms; in the case of a child, also look under Hyperactivity. Dosage: page 31.

KEY SYMPTOMS	REMEDY
Legs and arms are restless; heart pounding; jittery; hands and feet "go to sleep" easily; anxious; excited; "runs" hot and cold. *Worse:* nights	**Aconitum**
Nervousness affecting the heart, severe pounding of heart; headaches with dizziness and feeling dazed; anxious; whiny. *Worse:* in the evening, 3 to 4 A.M., warmth, summer *Better:* outdoors, in company	**Aethusa**
Nervous itching; skin is red with burning sensation; also nose itching—inside and out; physical restlessness; movement coordination is disturbed. *Worse:* nicotine, cold, thunderstorm, after a meal *Better:* slow movements	**Agarius**
Extremely sensitive, very exited; talks non-stop; constantly thinks about uncomfortable things; cries when listening to music; skin feels numb. Particularly for children and very thin people. *Worse:* in the morning, in warm rooms, around a stranger	**Ambra**
Nervous restlessness due to overwork and shock; does not talk about problems; wants to be alone, fear of public places; headaches	**Arnica**

with dizziness, nervous sharp chest pain.
Worse: touch, motion
Better: lying down

Extremely sensitive and impatient; overactive;   **Chamomilla**
quarrelsome; screams; many different physical
symptoms; intolerant to pain. Especially
for children.
Worse: evenings, nights, from touch, when angry,
from coffee
Better: warmth, alone

Painfully restless; talks constantly; can't   **Lachesis**
concentrate; often after being mentally
overloaded; suspicious; jealous; intolerant of
tight clothing; hot flashes; apprehensive.
Also in women during menopause.
Worse: sleep, warmth in any form
Better: menstruation, after a hot flash

Nervous restlessness before and after thunder-   **Natrum**
storms; heat, music; worry about the future.   **carbonicum**

Extreme physical discomfort; can't sit still;   **Rhus**
nervous skin rashes; joints and ligaments   **toxicodendron**
ache; headache with dizziness when getting
up in the morning.
Better: motion and walking

Nervous twitching of the corner of the   **Zincum**
mouth, feet tense before and during   **metallicum**
menstruation or menopause; backache;
shivers when feeling weak.
Worse: evening, nights, touch, fright
Better: motion

HYPERACTIVITY

Hyperactivity is a problem that most often afflicts children of kindergarten and grammar school age. Always take into consideration the basic constitution of the child and his or her present circumstances. Often hyperactivity occurs after there has been a severe infectious illness, particularly after a childhood illness that has been treated with antibiotics. When you find circumstances like these, seek the advice of your physician or homeopath. Hyperactivity can be a permanent condition and is accompanied by disturbed fine and gross motor activity and increased aggressiveness. Dosage: page 31.

KEY SYMPTOMS	REMEDY
Physically and mentally hyperactive; always in motion; always has new ideas; has little staying power; happy; quick learner; easily excited; laughs and cries at the time; heart is pounding. *Worse:* coffee, tea, chamomile tea; when exited, smells, noise, nights *Better:* warmth, lying down, licking/eating ice	**Coffea**
Extremely sensitive to all external stimuli; has stimulus overload; wants to do and take in everything at once; has little staying power; restless, fidgety, fragile, loves company; intelligent; imaginative. *Worse:* noise, light, smells, touch, twilight, thunderstorms, change in the weather *Better:* nights, cold food, outdoors, sleep	**Phosphorus**

MOOD SWINGS

Help is always needed when mood swings become problematic for the person who has them. Check also under the terms Irritability, Sadness, or Restlessness. In a case of sudden and extreme mood swings or when the complaints have existed for some time, always seek advice from your physician or homeopath. Dosage: page 31.

KEY SYMPTOMS	REMEDY
Nothing is right, always dissatisfied; unkind; morose; won't talk; sentimental; romantic with sudden ecstasy; everything affects the stomach. *Worse:* when addressed, paid attention to; touch	**Antimonium crudum**
Contradictory behavior, particularly in the case of overwork and worry; inappropriate laughing spells; rage against uninvolved persons; crying spells. *Worse:* when taking stimulants *Better:* warmth, moderate motion	**Ignatia**
Mood similar to "April weather"; shy, timid, gentle, helpful; irritated, suspicious, jealous, smug; crying for no apparent reason, laughing hysterically; in severe crisis, however, strong and forceful.	**Pulsatilla**

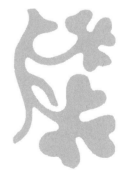

LACK OF CONCENTRATION AND POOR MEMORY

Lack of concentration and poor memory are a sign of mental exhaustion and overwork. They can also be caused by traumatic events and illnesses. If such an illness is due to anemia, a physician should do blood tests immediately, with particular emphasis on iron. (Iron deficiencies can't be treated with homeopathic remedies, only in combination with specific iron preparations.) In cases where complaints are severe and accompanied by episodes of confusion, seek advice from your physician or homeopath. Dosage: page 31.

KEY SYMPTOMS	REMEDY
Unable to find words, difficulty in comprehension, listless, apathetic. Particularly after sorrow, shock, overwork, during puberty.	**Acidum phosphoricum**
Lack of concentration and forgetfulness, causing an aversion to doing any mental activities; constantly using profanity; ravenous appetite.	**Anacardium carbonicum**
Forgetful, mentally weak; lack of self-confidence; aversion to strangers. Particularly for children and older people.	**Barium**
Head feels "empty" but confused, can't concentrate; headaches on the right side. Particularly in case of exhaustion after illness.	**Iridium**
General mental and emotional exhaustion, head "feels" numb, fear of failure, suspicious of conspiracy, melancholy.	**Kali bromatum**
Extreme forgetfulness due to weakness/exhaustion; makes writing mistakes; depressed.	**Lac caninum**

KEY SYMPTOMS	REMEDY
Poor memory, lack of concentration when under stress; makes writing and spelling mistakes; can't read own writing.	**Lycopodium**
General lack of motivation and poor memory; answers slowly; suspicious; fear of going insane.	**Mercurius solubilis**
Forgetful, very sleepy; moves as if in a dream; often after emotional shock and when being lovesick.	**Nux moschata**
Forgetful; lack of concentration; poor coordination due to exhaustion; feels as if "born tired"; often headaches/migraine on the left side.	**Onosmodium**
Easily distracted, extremely sensitive to external stimuli; little staying power.	**Phosphorus**
Perception slowed, memory reduced; depressed to apathetic; often with anemia.	**Plumbum acetum**
Extreme forgetfulness, mentally sluggish, delusional; extremely self-absorbed.	**Sulfur**

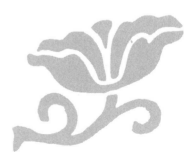

INSOMNIA

Insomnia usually is the result of fear, worry, grief, being overly tired, over-worked, or sick, but also can occur after having eaten disagreeable food. Therefore check also under the respective terms, including Restlessness. What follows here is only a brief list of symptoms that are characteristic of some of the reasons for insomnia, including the situations in which they usually occur. If insomnia has been going on for some time, conventional sleeping aids have been tried, and the remedies listed here have brought no relief, see your physician or homeopath immediately. Dosage: page 31.

KEY SYMPTOMS	REMEDY
Scary dreams, distressing nightmares; abrupt awakening from sleep; insomnia affecting seniors; after emotional shock and fever.	**Aconitum**
Anxious, restless, confusing dreams; tired and sleepy in the morning. Particularly in sensitive children and seniors. *Better:* warm room	**Alumina**
Tired but can't go to sleep because of worries; has to get up and walk around; muscles twitching during sleep; limbs are cold or numb.	**Ambra**
Difficulty falling asleep before a test or important appointments; always expects the worst; scary dreams; exhausted in the morning.	**Argentum nitricum**
Can't sleep due to being over-tired, restless; exhausted; scary dreams, waking up between 2 and 3 o'clock in the morning. *Better:* sleeping on a softer surface	**Arnica**

KEY SYMPTOMS	REMEDY
Difficulty falling asleep due to worry and fear of failure; awakens after nightmares; often physically totally exhausted; is mentally overactive.	**Arsenicum album**
Restless, screams, grinds teeth; startled when falling asleep and during sleep; bothered by pulsating sensation in the blood vessels; particularly when there is fever and/or headaches.	**Belladonna**
Can't fall asleep due to worries at work or from exciting bedtime reading; awakened by scary dreams.	**Bryonia**
Won't fall asleep until the early morning hours; awakens frequently from the most minuscule noises, has constantly reappearing unpleasant thoughts; grinds teeth, chews; for children's nightmares. *Worse:* cold, full moon	**Calcarea carbonica**
Tired, unable to fall asleep; extremely hot; particularly after angry confrontations and coffee; muscle cramps and rheumatism.	**Chamomilla**
Can't fall asleep even if overly tired; yawning spasms; particularly because of lack of sleep, night work, or nursing.	**Cocculus**
Total mental/physical over-stimulation, can't fall asleep; awakens constantly; hears every sound; particularly when overly tired. Too much coffee, tea, or chamomile tea.	**Coffea**
Light, restless sleep before a test and important appointments; can't fall asleep, is thinking constantly.	**Gelsemium**

KEY SYMPTOMS	REMEDY
Muscle twitching while falling asleep; light sleep with long and heavy dreams; arms itching; intense yawning; occurs after grief and worry.	**Ignatia**
Sleeplessness because of grief and worry; fear of failure; nightmares; grinding teeth; sleep walking.	**Kali bromatum**
Wide awake in the evening; works till midnight; tired and still can't sleep; light, restless sleep. *Worse:* warmth, in the morning	**Lachesis**
Dreaming about accidents; dazed during the day.	**Lycopodium**
Can't fall asleep due to worries and having been offended; twitching muscles during sleep; dreams of robbery.	**Natrum chloratum**
Thoughts revolve around work and business.	**Nux vomica**
Restless, children or seniors waking up often.	**Passiflora**
Waking up constantly; falls asleep late and tired when waking up; very tired after a meal; hungry during the night.	**Phosphorus**
Wide awake in the evening; very tired in the afternoon; trouble falling asleep; wakes up before midnight, often hands are crossed over head or stomach.	**Pulsatilla**
Totally exhausted; falls asleep late; wakes up frequently; thinks somebody has been calling; insomnia during the early morning hours.	**Sepia**

KEY SYMPTOMS	REMEDY
Late falling asleep, wakes up before midnight and then can't go back to sleep; severe perspiration of the head; sleepwalking.	**Silicea**
Light, drowsy sleep; wakes up frequently (like a cat); talks in sleep; needs lots of pillows; pushes feet out from under the covers.	**Sulfur**
Nervous sleep with muscle cramps and itchy skin, worsens upon waking up; vivid dreams. *Worse:* valerian	**Valeriana**

CHAPTER 2

Headaches and Other General Discomforts

BASIC INFORMATION

Headaches and other similar discomforts, such as exhaustion, tiredness, and distinct reactions to changes in the weather, are always a sign that the body's overall mental/emotional/physical balance has become disturbed. The causes for this condition are many, and several factors usually contribute to a given situation. In most cases, an imbalance is related to working and living habits whose unhealthy effects we tend to admit only grudgingly. Causes such as these include what we eat and the demands we make on the energy available to us at any given time. The treatment of acute complaints with homeopathic remedies is intended to reestablish the mental/emotional/physical balance of the patient and, most importantly in the case of headaches, to regulate the condition of the blood vessels in the head. This will untimately reduce painful and uncomfortable symptoms.

In the long run, however, homeopathic remedies will not be able to overcome the effects of an unhealthy lifestyle and the constant self-inflicted overburdening of one's available energies. People who are constantly weakening their vitality should not be surprised when alarm signals like headaches and discomforts become more shrill, but they should be aware that there might be long-term severe and possibly irreversible organic illnesses in the making. All those who are suffering from constant headaches and other disturbances in their overall well-being should seek the advice of an experienced homeopath.

In this chapter, we are only discussing acute headaches and general discomforts that are not related to those illnesses that need medical attention. We will not discuss, for example, high blood pressure, metabolic illnesses, wounds due to injuries, or acute infections. Since the list of remedies for headaches is very long, we have organized headaches according to their trigger mechanism. An overlapping of remedies is very well possible. For instance, a remedy that is listed under Migraine may also be listed under the so-called simple headache, if the characteristics of the symptoms associated with it are analogous. Also, due to lack of space, the descriptions of symptoms have been limited to mentioning only the type and location of the pain and the modality. For that reason, before finally deciding on a remedy, it is essential that you compare the complaints and the condition against the mental/emotional character of the symptoms discussed in Chapter 3. If the characteristic symptoms are not listed, choose a different remedy.

When to See Your Physician

Seek medical help immediately in any of the following situations:

- severe headaches with high fever, nausea, vomiting, and a stiff neck
  NOTE: In the case of a child, also during the course of a childhood disease, like measles, mumps, and scarlet fever.
- suddenly appearing, severe headaches with signs of paralysis, vision problems and when a person is losing consciousness (emergency room)
- sudden, severe headaches after having taken a medication
- after head injuries

If you have already taken conventional pain medication for some time, see an experienced homeopath. Original symptoms may have been covered over or altered by conventional pain medicine, so a long-term, multiple-stage treatment might be necessary to achieve relief. This holds true especially for a patient suffering from neuralgic head and facial pain or from migraine.

HEADACHES FROM OVERWORK AND EXHAUSTION

Acute headaches are usually due to mental and/or physical stress, over-work, eyestrain, or working under a deadline, etc. They most often occur in combination with lack of sleep. IMPORTANT: If you are suffering from these types of headache, reduce and/or reorganize your work load, take regular breaks, and get a sufficient amount of sleep.

KEY SYMPTOMS	REMEDY
Pain pressing like a weight from the back of the head all the way to the forehead; dizzy when getting up; particularly due to emotional but often also mental overexertion; totally apathetic. Often during puberty. *Worse:* in the morning, motion, speaking, light, cold weather, warm rooms *Better:* bed rest, warmth (compresses), fresh air, liquid diet, given comfort	**Acidum phosphoricum**
Total exhaustion due to overwork; bursting pain that often starts at the neck; fatigue from any type of effort; everything is too much; tired during the day, wide awake or adventurous at night. Often for school children. *Worse:* in the morning, warm rooms *Better:* cool fresh air, quiet, lying down	**Acidum picrinicum**
Bursting pain as if hit by a pole; feeling as if the head is in a vise; after mental strain; lack of concentration; forgetful; dizziness; very sensitive; suspicious. *Better:* from eating	**Anacardium**
Stubborn "school headaches" in children, on the top of the head; makes excessive demands; suffers from lack of sleep. *Worse:* fresh air, change of weather *Better:* eating, midday nap, lying down	**Calcarea phosphorica**

KEY SYMPTOMS	REMEDY

Pounding, pulsating pain at the temples, as
if the head is going to burst; skin on top of
the head feels numb; physically exhausted;
mentally alert but can't concentrate; often
due to anemia.
Worse: touch, noise/excitement, cold air, draft
Better: pressure, gentle motion

China

Oppressive, thumping pain in the forehead
and neck; nausea; dizziness; dazed; mentally
overworked; lack of sleep due to night work.
Worse: motion, driving a car; eating, excitement
Better: lying down, a short nap

Cocculus

Stabbing, pounding, pulsating pain, also
at the back of the head; when in pain, face
reddens and feet are cold; hair roots are painful,
keeps hair loose; often due to anemia.
Worse: after any type of effort, including mental
Better: walking about slowly, after getting up
in the morning, lying down

Ferrum metallicum

Stress headaches due to mental overexertion;
too much nicotine, alcohol; under time
pressures, troubled, chilled; choleric;
pedantic; overly sensitive.
Worse: in the morning, cold, draft, sun, noise, light
Better: warm room, lying down, a short nap

Nux vomica

Dull pain from the neck all the way to the
forehead; anxiously despondent; feels small
and overtaxed. Occurs in children.
Worse: motion, noise
Better: wrapped up warmly, pressure

Silicea

NERVOUS HEADACHES

Nervous headaches are often triggered by (repressed) irritation, anger, rage, feelings of frustration, and stage fright, as well as time pressure, loud noises, and one's generally being overly sensitive. Those who experience frequent bouts of nervous headaches should try take take more time for themselves in order to regain their sense of balance. IMPORTANT: Avoid coffee, tea, alcohol, and TV-watching!

KEY SYMPTOMS	REMEDY
Piercing pain inside the head, often also in the right or left temple; nausea with vomiting; dizziness; chills easily; very impulsive but also very anxious. *Worse:* lack of sleep, mental strain *Better:* pressure, cold (compresses)	**Argentum nitricum**
Severe pain in the front of the head, reaching all the way to the back of the head, neck, and shoulders; nervous exhaustion; everything is too much; morose; wants to be left alone. *Worse:* in the morning, motion of any kind *Better:* rest/quiet, pressure	**Bryonia**
Pounding pain, often one-sided with face flushed on one side; overly sensitive; over-reacting; impatient and angry. *Worse:* lack of sleep, coffee, when angry, when given words of comfort *Better:* cold food and drinks, out driving in car	**Chamomilla**
Stabbing, pulsating pain (like nail pounding), all senses are overstimulated; after positive surprises; wound up mentally and physically; can't sleep. *Worse:* noise, light, motion *Better:* rest, cold compresses	**Coffea**

KEY SYMPTOMS	REMEDY

Stabbing, pounding pain that moves all the time or feels like nails are pounded into the temple; vomiting; strong urge to urinate; very emotional and contradictory; sick with anger; worried.
Worse: in the morning, coffee, nicotine, smoke (tobacco), light, conversation
Better: lying down, food, sighing

Ignatia

Headaches from stress (being under time pressure and mental overwork); often accompanied by problems with digestion; choleric; pedantic; overly sensitive.
Worse: in the morning, cold, sun
Better: warm room, lying down, short nap

Nux vomica

Burning, piercing pain in the forehead, often above one eye; nausea; very excitable but little staying power; anxious; annoyed. Especially found in children.
Worse: in the morning, when excited
Better: when given comfort, cold food, sleep, cold air

Phosphorus

Moving, piercing pain in the forehead and above the eyes or with a feeling that the head seems to be bursting, often on the right side; dizziness; very gentle but moody; dissatisfied.
Worse: in the morning, warmth, mental strain
Better: when given comfort, fresh air, motion

Pulsatilla D12

Severe, pulsating pain, one-sided in the temple and one eye; severe tearing; starts in the morning, is worst at noon, ends in the early evening; all senses are overly sensitive; irrational fears.
Worse: motion, noises
Better: lying down

Spigelia

Severe attack of pain in the forehead;   **Valeriana**
piercing pressure; internal restlessness;
lack of concentration; jumpy. Particularly
for those who work mentally.
Worse: rest, in the evening, strain
Better: motion, rubbing

HEADACHES DUE TO MUSCLE TENSION

A frequent reason for headaches, particularly for people who work sitting down, is muscle tension in the neck and shoulder area. The tension reduces the flow of blood and thereby oxygen to the head, the product of which is pain and other complaints. Those suffering from this type of headache frequently should check their work place according to ergo-dynamic criteria. For example, they should make sure the height of the chair is correct and notice the demands that their activities make on their posture. But they should also keep in mind other tensions and pressures and consider if they have taken on too many responsibilities.

KEY SYMPTOMS   **REMEDY**

Heaviness in the back of the head and the neck,   **Acidum**
overwork, worry; piercing pain; any effort is   **picrinicum**
too much; tired during the day, awake at night.
Worse: in the morning, warm room
Better: cool temperatures, fresh air, rest,
lying down

Heavy pain from the neck, up to above the   **Cimicifuga**
eyes; top of the head seems to burst; neck and   **racemosa**
shoulders are very tense; very nervous.
Worse: mental effort, cold weather, menopause
Better: warmth

Heavy, pounding pain in the forehead and neck,   **Cocculus**
difficulty holding head up; dizziness; nausea;
overwork (night work), stress, and worry.

KEY SYMPTOMS	REMEDY

Worse: driving a car, lying on back, coffee
Better: lying down, short nap

Dull, heavy pain from the top of the head to the shoulders; feeling of having a vise around the head or wearing a hat; neck feels squeezed. Particularly occurs with stage fright and test anxiety. *Worse:* in the morning, warmth *Better:* after urinating	**Gelsemium**

Stabbing pain, often in the back of the head and above one eye; severe tension in the neck and shoulders; mentally overworked, under time pressure; too much nicotine, coffee, and alcohol. *Worse:* in the morning, draft, cold, sun *Better:* warm room, lying down, short nap	**Nux vomica**

HEADACHES FROM HANGOVERS

These headaches typically occur after an all-night party, too much nicotine, alcohol, and food.

KEY SYMPTOMS	REMEDY
Numbing, dull headache and nausea after too much wine consumption, particularly from sour wine and sour food. *Worse:* in the morning, sun, warmth *Better:* fresh air, cool air	**Antimonium crudum**
Roaring headaches; nausea; dizziness; digestive problems; too much nicotine, alcohol, and rich food; lack of sleep.	**Nux vomica**
As for *Nux vomica* (main remedy), but for introverted, sensitive people. Especially for those bothered by smells and tobacco smoke.	**Ignatia**

NEURALGIA OF THE HEAD AND FACE

These headaches are caused by painful stimulation of specific nerves in the head, particularly the trigeminus nerve. They are often the result of exposure to wind or are brought on by a change in the weather. This pain can be precipitated by emotional or physical stress, dental problems, and can result from ear and eye problems (also check under that category). In some cases the causes are unknown. These headaches often affect only one side of the head. Make sure that your physician has ruled out any possible organic causes.

KEY SYMPTOMS	REMEDY
Severe, cutting pain with feelings of numbness and tingling; often caused by cold winds, including drafts while driving and open windows; the painful area of the face is also flushed and swollen; very agitated, anxious. *Worse:* in the evening, at night *Better:* rest, warmth	**Aconitum D12**
Stabbing, burning pain as if poked with a hot needle; also numbness and tingling; face is cold and pale; very restless and anxious, pedantic. *Worse:* at midnight, in cold *Better:* warmth (compresses)	**Arsenicum album D12**
Pulsating, pounding, stabbing pain, usually on one side only, radiates into ears and teeth; painful area is flushed and hot, the other half of the face is pale; general oversensitivity. *Worse:* nights, stress, wind, coffee *Better:* motion, driving	**Chamomilla**
Splitting, heavy pain; usually on the right temple, radiating into the upper jaw; often concentrated above the right eye; intense tearing; forehead very sensitive to pressure.	**Chelidonium majus**

KEY SYMPTOMS	REMEDY

Worse: early morning, motion, touch
Better: eating

Severe, one-sided pain in the upper and lower jaw: stabbing or numbing; starts in the morning and after breakfast.
Worse: on vacation, weekends, resting, fresh air
Better: activity

Iris

Cramplike pain in short, lightning attacks; often one-sided from the face down into the neck; face often flushed; general exhaustion.
Worse: cold, cold water, touch, motion
Better: warmth, pressure

Magnesium phosphoricum

Pounding pain moving from neck across the center of the skull to the right eye; usually starting early in the morning; returning periodically every several days. Particularly during menopause.
Worse: noise, light, sun
Better: lying down, sleeping, eating

Sanguinara canadensis

Severe, pulsating, burning pain, often into the neck and shoulders; also in the lower jaw or the eyes, causing severe tearing; often during damp or cold weather; starts in the morning; is worst by noon, ends in the evening.
Worse: motion, noise
Better: quiet, lying down

Spigelia

MIGRAINE HEADACHES

Migraine headaches are caused by a sudden contraction of the blood vessels in the head. Symptoms include vision problems, numbness in the area of the head or the limbs; a feeling of being dazed; nausea and vomiting. Because of the consequent dilation of the blood vessels, severe, often one-sided, headaches set in that can be accompanied by dizziness, further nausea and vomiting, and severe sensitivity to light. Various triggers may set off a reaction: emotional stress, alcohol, nicotine, medication, hormonal imbalance, cocoa products, nuts, cheeses, citrus fruits. The diagnosis of migraine must always be made by a physician. In cases of severe and frequently recurring migraine headaches, always consult your physician or an experienced homeopath. IMPORTANT: The following remedies might be able to shorten the duration of an attack but the complaints will not be healed immediately.

KEY SYMPTOMS	REMEDY
Gray spots in front of your eyes; excruciating pain in the right temple and the right side of the face; pain appears and disappears suddenly; starts in the morning, is worst at midday, gets better by evening. *Worse:* mental stress, smells *Better:* wrapping the head tightly, quiet	**Argentum nitricum**
Brief periods of vision problems, sparkles or dark spots in front of the eyes; one-sided headaches with feelings of seething pressure in the blood vessels or bitter cold in the head. *Worse:* cold, wetness, stress	**Calcarea carbonica**
A flickering/sparkles in front of the eyes, dizziness when turning; stabbing pain in the temples and forehead; starts in the morning; individual is exhausted, touchy, sad. *Worse:* during difficult menstruation, lying on the painful side, lying on the back, outdoors *Better:* being alone, warmth	**Cyclamen**

KEY SYMPTOMS	REMEDY
Blurred vision; crossed eyes; double vision; dizziness. Severe pain starts in the neck and goes from the back of the head to the left eye; face is hot and flushed; extreme exhaustion. *Worse:* in the morning, motion, damp weather, fog, sun, stress *Better:* with head elevated, urinating	**Gelsemium**
Blurred vision; pounding headache from the back of the head to the eyes; nausea; sour, bitter-tasting vomit that does not bring relief; often on weekends or on vacation, or after mental stress. *Worse:* quiet, cold air *Better:* motion	**Iris**
Vision distorted by zigzaging lines; briefly losing sight; pounding pain, mostly on right side; face is pale; anemic; introvert; unforgiving. *Worse:* about 10 A.M., noise, motion, when comforted *Better:* evenings, quiet, when alone, lying down	**Natrum chloratum**
Difficulty with vision; everything seems to be larger than it really is; extreme pain, as if a nail is being pounded into head; starts at the left side; pressure at the center of the head; nervous twitch of the upper lip; vertebrae in neck make cracking sound in morning. *Worse:* beginning in morning, into afternoon *Better:* evening, rubbing	**Niccolum**
Blurred vision, often due to overly stressed eyes; squeezing pain from the back of the head to the temple and eye sockets, usually on the left side; dizziness; coordination of movements disturbed. *Worse:* in the dark, when lying down *Better:* lying on back, eating, sleeping	**Onosmodium**

SENSITIVITY TO CHANGES IN THE WEATHER

Some people seem to have almost "allergic" reactions to changes in the weather; they are often able to tell when a change is approaching by the headaches they experience or by rheumatic complaints, extreme tiredness and increased nervousness. Being sensitive to changes in the weather is without a doubt bothersome and uncomfortable, but the complaints are not equal to being sick. However, those who suffer from massive complaints should consult an experienced homeopath.

KEY SYMPTOMS	REMEDY
Headaches at the seams of the skull; sensitive hair roots; rheumatic complaints; previous bone fractures are painful. *Worse:* damp/cold weather, melting snow *Better:* warm and sunny weather	**Calcarea phosphorica**
Piercing, burning, dull pain in the forehead like having a "board nailed to the head"; in cases of sudden temperature changes; cold nights in the summer; damp cold. *Better:* warm weather in the summertime	**Dulcamara**
Stabbing, piercing pain that seems to spilt apart the whole head; often one-sided; after being exposed to drafty, cold, dry, stormy weather. *Better:* when it begins to rain, damp warmth, warm rooms	**Hepar sulfuris**
Pounding headache, head feels hot and heavy; dizziness; extremely nervous; sudden onset in hot weather and sunshine; also in the spring; can't tolerate tight clothing. *Worse:* taking a nap in the middle of the day	**Lachesis**
Dull headache with nausea; starts before the weather turns hot and sunny; also before a	**Natrum carbonicum**

thunderstorm; summer heat causes great
weakness.
Worse: mental stress

Rheumatic pain; feels every change from dry to damp weather; pain in the back of the neck, accompanied by dizziness; particularly in damp indoor places; fog. *Better:* warmth, dry air	**Natrum sulfuricum**

Neuralgic pain in the shoulder; stiff neck;
headaches; person frequently shivers, even
when it is warm.
Worse: humid/cold weather, cold wind, draft
Better: warmth

Nux vomica

Rheumatic complaints; skin is "crawling" and
numb; sciatica pain; heavy head or headaches
as if a board has been nailed to the forehead,
dizziness when getting up; brought on particularly
by sudden changes in the weather; in the fall;
being chilled after perspiring by exposure to
cold winds.

**Rhus
toxicodendron**

Oppressive headaches that go from the back of
the head to the forehead; neuralgic facial pain
and toothache; old scars are hurting; sciatic
complaints; reduced motivation; constantly cold.
Worse: when weather changes to cold

Silicea

TIREDNESS, WEAKNESS, AND FATIGUE

Complaints of this type of intense fatigue are usually the result of work overload and extraordinary stress—pregnancy, after a birth and subsequent nursing, moving—and other types of changes at work and at home. The "battery" is simply empty. Reduce the amount of daily chores, take a break, relax, and eat healthy food in order to recharge your energies. In addition to the remedies listed on pages 56 and 57, the following remedies also may be helpful. IMPORTANT: If complaints have been around for some time or if they are getting worse, it is essential that you see your physician.

KEY SYMPTOMS	REMEDY
Total physical and emotional/mental exhaustion; feeling beat up; insomnia.	**Arnica**
Extreme physical weakness; constantly cold; fear of a total breakdown or illness.	**Arsenicum album D12**
Extreme perspiration with only minimum exertion; damp/cold feet; feels cold.	**Calcarea carbonica**
Nervous and fragile due to mental/emotional stress; shy; talks little; frightened; headaches accompanied by dizziness; diminishing vision; ravenous for sweets and for sour-tasting foods. Particularly for young people. *Worse:* mornings, cold, exertion *Better:* warmth, quiet	**Kali phosphoricum**
Nervous exhaustion due to overstimulation; sudden bouts of weakness with perspiration and fear.	**Phosphorus**
Total exhaustion due to overwork; dizziness and bouts of weakness almost like fainting. Particularly for working mothers and women.	**Sepia**

CHAPTER 3

Respiratory Problems

VIRAL INFECTION (FLU)

Often accompanied by fever, viral infections commonly known as the flu are a seasonal occurrence. Many times they start out with nonspecific symptoms, like exhaustion, aching head and joints, and fever; later, all the typical complaints of a cold are added (see also under that subject). The following remedies have proven to be effective in the early stages of a viral infection. But seek medical attention in more advanced and severe situations where the fever is above 102° F/39° C, where heart and circulatory problems occur, or where a stiff neck and severe headaches are experienced.

NOTE: A viral infection always affects the whole system, including muscle tissues; that's why the muscles and joints tend to ache. Always make sure that you allow the body to heal; this means, stay in bed. It is the only way to avoid severe complications, like heart and circulatory problems. After recovery, a homeopathic constitutional therapy is highly recommended.

KEY SYMPTOMS	REMEDY
Turbulent beginning; result of cold, dry wind often from East, also draft while driving a car; scared/angry; shivers, usually starting at midnight; nightmares; afraid of death; extreme restlessness; skin hot and dry; face flushed when lying down, pale when sitting up; extremely thirsty for cold water. *Worse:* evening, warm rooms, in dry winds *Better:* after a bout of perspiration	**Aconitum D12*/****
Sudden onset; pounding headaches make every movement painful; pupils dilated, eyes red; face flushes to a bright, dark red, with heat, perspiration; the whole body is feverish while feet are often cold; mouth is dry without	**Belladonna D6***

*One standard dose every 30 minutes, 4 times maximum.
**If experienced, can use 1 or 2 doses at C30 potency.

being thirsty; extremely sensitive or numb.
Worse: cold, motion
Better: warmth (warm bed), quiet

Starts out slowly; the whole body feels   **Eupatorium**
beaten up; joints seem twisted; constant   **perfoliatum D6**
backache; pounding, bursting headache;
face is flushed, hot, but shows no perspiration;
fever is highest in early afternoon; shivering
fever at night and in the morning; wants to
drink cold water; vomiting after shivers; painful
cough, clutching hands to chest.
Worse: motion

Starts slowly; often people—children—who   **Ferrum**
get tired quickly, but stay mentally alert; dull   **phosphoricum**
headaches; face alternately flushed and pale;   **D6 or D12**
tendency to get nosebleeds and inner ear
infection with pounding pain that seems to
appear in waves; fever rather low; night
perspiration; either very thirsty or not at all;
complaints are viewed as light, wants to get
out of bed.
Worse: early mornings

A cold is coming on but remains latent; first   **Gelsemium D12**
complaints usually two to three days after
having caught a cold; in the beginning often
severe shivering—the teeth rattle; wants to
be held; followed by fluctuating fever, highest
around 3 P.M. face is swollen and flushed;
runny nose; dazed; head and joints ache; too
weak to talk, wants to be left alone; hands and
feet are cold.
Worse: afternoons, stress
Better: fresh air, after urinating, coffee and tea

SORE THROAT

A sore throat usually involves difficulty swallowing and inflammation (look for redness) in the tonsils and throat tissue. In cases of hoarseness and cough, see Laryngitis. Though primarily due to an acute viral infection of the throat and tonsils (it can be bacterial in some cases), a sore throat is also often accompanied by a cold. In the presence of a high fever (102° F/39° C) and pus (white stipples), see your physician immediately.

KEY SYMPTOMS	REMEDY
Sudden onset; reason: cold/dry wind, often East winds; also draft while driving in a car; throat feels tight, burning pain; thirsty for water only; fever climbs fast; skin hot and dry. *Worse:* cold, wind, motion *Better:* rest	**Aconitum D12***
Stabbing pain in the throat as if injured by a splinter, also burning pain; tissue in the throat very red, glassy, or covered with mucus; fever above 101° F/38° C; not thirsty. *Worse:* warmth *Better:* cold, cold drinks, cool fresh air	**Apis mellifica D6**
Severe, stabbing, burning pain in the throat; reason: damp/cold weather; throat is dry, must swallow constantly; fever; skin is hot, red, and sweaty; irritating sneezing when swallowing food and drink; barely thirsty. *Worse:* after midnight, cold, talking *Better:* rest/quiet	**Dulcamara D6**

*One dose every 30 minutes, 4 times maximum.

KEY SYMPTOMS	REMEDY
Pain in the throat wanders from the left to the right side, radiating into the ears; throat and tonsils are bluish-red; highly sensitive to touch; can't stand anything tight around the neck; highly uncomfortable in warm rooms; pain aggravated by hot drinks. *Worse:* warmth, stale air, after sleeping *Better:* fresh air	**Lachesis D12**
Dry, sore throat; increasingly scratchy; throat feels tight; pain starts on the right side and moves to the left; can barely swallow; demands for something warm to drink; dark circles under the eyes; grayish-yellow face color; stubborn; easily exhausted. *Worse:* in the afternoon, warm bed, cold drinks *Better:* warm drinks, fresh air	**Lycopodium D12**
Sore throat, increasingly scratchy; itches when waking up; has tendency to catch a cold in cool weather; is easily cold, usually has something wrapped around the throat; is angry about the symptoms, impatient; unkind. *Worse:* in the morning, cold, mental stress *Better:* in the evening, rest, short nap	**Nux vomica D12**
Sore, hot throat; feeling of tightness; pain radiates into the ears; tonsils and tissues in the throat and are dark red to bluish; often only on the right side; mucus formation at the base of the tongue; must swallow constantly; lymph nodes are swollen. *Worse:* warm drinks, warmth (in bed) *Better:* cold drinks	**Phytolacca D6**

TONSILLITIS

Tonsillitis, in most cases, is a bacterial infection of the tonsils and progresses in different stages. Self-treatment is suggested only for those who have already used homeopathy successfully and only when the illness is in its beginning stages with complaints that appear suddenly.

IMPORTANT: If the remedies listed here do not improve condition within the first 24 hours, or if the patient's fever is already high (102° F/39° C) and accompanied by severe pain on both sides of the throat; if swallowing is painful; or if the tonsils are already covered with white pus (white spots and the person's breath has an especially bad odor), medical treatment must be sought immediately.

KEY SYMPTOMS   **REMEDY**

Stabbing, burning throat pain, tonsils are   **Apis mellifica D6**
severely swollen and covered with a glossy
layer of mucus; person is extremely sensitive to
touch; cannot stand anything tight; shivering and
not thirsty; fever highest in the late afternoon;
little urine, of dark color.
Worse: warmth (including a shawl around the
neck), warm drink
Better: fresh, cool air
IMPORTANT: Every *Apis* tonsillitis must be closely
watched. Check with your physician, even in the
early stages. Drink plenty of fluids!

Throat feels as if swollen/tied shut, barely   **Belladonna D6***
able to swallow; tonsils severely swollen;
mouth is dry; tongue dry, shiny, raspberry-
red; pupils dilated; conjunctiva is red; skin is
tomato-red, hot, and steaming; need for
something cold to drink, even if it hurts to
swallow; takes liquid in small sips.
Worse: cold drinks, cold, swallowing, speaking
Better: covered with warm blankets

*One dose every 30 minutes, 4 times maximum.

KEY SYMPTOMS	REMEDY
Stabbing pain, radiating into the ears; tonsils bright red; right side often worse; mouth is dry; tongue is red only on the sides and the tip; slimy covering at the base of the tongue; palate is dark red; fever without perspiration, and only increasing slowly; head is hot, body cold; feels very weak—beat up; wants to move about which, however, brings no relief. *Worse:* warm liquids, solid food, during the night *Better:* cold fluids	**Phytolacca D6**

LARYNGITIS

General laryngitis symptoms are a scratchy throat, hoarseness, and a cough. Often an acute viral or bacterial infection of the larynx, it can also be caused by the irritation of air pollution. In cases of a high fever (102° F/ 39° C), severe difficulty breathing, and pus formation (white spots in the throat), see your physician immediately. ATTENTION: Small children in rare cases might, during the night, have attacks of croup-like coughing with breathing difficulty. Call your physician immediately if this should occur.

KEY SYMPTOMS	REMEDY
Suddenly develops shivers because of a cold, dry wind, draft from driving a car, or becoming frightened; has anxious feelings and nightmares, particularly children; skin is hot and red; face flushed when lying down, pale when sitting up; throat feels like being strangled, has a short, dry cough. *Worse:* cold, wind, motion *Better:* rest/quiet	**Aconitum D12***

*Depending on severity, l dose every 15 to 60 minutes but no more than a total of 5 doses; if experienced, 1 or 2 at C30.

KEY SYMPTOMS	REMEDY
Burning pain in the throat; spells of dry cough with breathing difficulty; completely hoarse in the morning, better after coughing; has nosebleeds. *Worse:* cold, wetness, lying down, sleep *Better:* warmth, quiet, fresh air	**Ammonium carbonicum D6**
Sudden onset of hoarseness and scratchy throat; often after voice has been overused; voice gives out or has temporary loss of voice (often for singers, teachers, trainers/coaches). *Worse:* warm rooms *Better:* warm drinks	**Arum triphyllum D6**
Sudden, violent onset of pain with high fever; a burning in the throat; skin is hot and sweaty; face is bright red; wants to stay under the bed covers in spite of being hot; swallowing is painful; very thirsty for something cold; spasms of dry cough. Great children's remedy. *Worse:* nights, cold, talking *Better:* rest/quiet	**Belladonna D6***
Hoarseness in the morning due to dry, cold weather/wind; mucus is difficult to cough up; drops of urine escape when coughing; throat is dry and painful. *Worse:* dry/cold weather, dry/hot weather *Better:* when able to cough up mucus, after drinking cold fluids	**Causticum D12**
Painful swelling of the lymph nodes, very sensitive to touch; attacks of painful cough with breathing difficulty; bad breath. *Worse:* cold, in the early morning hours *Better:* moist warmth	**Hepar sulfuris D4 or D6**

*One dose every 30 minutes, but only for 2 hours.

76

KEY SYMPTOMS	REMEDY
Burning pain, particularly when swallowing and coughing; hoarseness, hollow-sounding; sometimes throat bleeds; wants something cold to drink but obvious worsening when exposed to external cold; afraid of thunderstorms. Particularly for singers.	**Phosphorus D12**
Hoarse and painful when swallowing; breathing difficulty; must clear throat constantly; cough is short and dry; is fearful; has swollen lymph nodes that are very sensitive to touch. *Worse:* external heat, motion, nights, after midnight *Better:* cold, eating, warm liquids	**Spongia D6**

BRONCHIAL COUGH

A bronchial cough often develops from a cough that was due to a cold (see Laryngitis). The cause of this ailment is also a viral (but can be bacterial) infection of the bronchial tubes, yet sometimes it is due to irritation from air pollution. Quite often these symptoms are chronic. Self-treatment in an acute case should only be administered by an experienced lay person. In case of high fever (102° F/39° C), see your physician immediately. ATTENTION: Measles, whooping cough, scarlet fever, and chicken pox can start out as a bronchial infection.

KEY SYMPTOMS	REMEDY
Raging cough with a feeling of suffocation; extreme amount of white, thick mucus that is difficult to expectorate; extreme exhaustion; breathing difficulty; pale complexion; nausea. A particularly suitable remedy for children and older people. *Worse:* nights (3 A.M.), lying down, damp/warm rooms	**Antimonium tartaricum D6**

KEY SYMPTOMS	REMEDY
Dry cough with stabbing chest pain; clutches chest when coughing; very sensitive to motion; thirsty, drinks a lot of liquid at once. *Worse:* motion, talking, change from warm to cold *Better:* quiet	**Bryonia D6**
A choking, cramp-like cough during the night and upon waking up; mucus expectorated is thick, clear, and stringy; coughing spells while brushing teeth. *Worse:* touch, stress, tight clothing, warm drinks *Better:* cold drinks, cool air	**Coccus cacti D6**
Dry, cramp-like coughing spells with attacks that follow each other quickly, particularly during the night; often accompanied by mucus draining from the nose; extremely weak after a coughing attack; very sensitive to cold air, breathes through a cloth; pulls blanket over the head. *Worse:* cold *Better:* warm rooms	**Corallium rubrum D6**
Dry, low, cramp-like cough, particularly during the night; short, severe attacks with fear of suffocation and vomiting, face turns blue-red; swollen blood vessels in the head; frequent vomiting; clutches chest during coughing spells; tendency of nosebleeds. *Worse:* after midnight, talking, singing, laughing, drinking, warmth	**Drosera D6**
Exhausting, cramp-like cough with fear of suffocation and rattling sounds in the bronchial tubes; mucus is thick, almost impossible to expectorate; wheezing cough; cramps when stretching; vomiting and nose-	**Ipecacuanha D6**

bleeding after a coughing spell; dark circles
under the eyes; pale complexion.
Worse: motion
Better: cold drinks

Acute cough due to a cold that has settled   **Pulsatilla D12**
in the throat; loose mucus; urine drips when
coughing; easily feels cold but can't handle
warmth.
Worse: in the evening, nights, warm/humid
weather
Better: in the morning, fresh air, outside

Exhausting coughing spells due to the feeling   **Rumex crispus D6**
of being tickled with a feather; often due to
cold air; dry cough after awakening in the
morning, in the evening when lying down,
and when eating; urge to urinate after a
coughing spell; frequent sneezing with pain
in the chest; wants to wrap the head in
something warm.
Worse: cold air, just before midnight and
between 2 and 4 A.M.
Better: in the morning

COLDS

A cold is characterized by inflammation of the inside of the nose and
sinuses and is usually caused by a virus. The reason we get colds is usually because of a general weakness of the immune system. Simple cold
symptoms could also be the early signs of a full-blown viral infection; if
there is fever, look instead under that subject. Complication due to a subsequent bacterial infection is not unusual (see also Sinus Infections and
Earaches). ATTENTION: Childhood diseases like measles and scarlet fever
often start out with an acute cold.

KEY SYMPTOMS	REMEDY
Painful, runny cold; nose and upper lip often are sore; foul-smelling mucus; in the beginning severe sneezing ; very restless and anxious, can't lie still. *Worse:* fresh air, cold *Better:* warmth	**Arsenicum album D12**
Painful runny cold; nose is sore; rubs nose until it bleeds; runny nose but still all stuffed up; breathes through the mouth. *Worse:* in the morning, warmth, lying down	**Arum triphyllum**
Painful, runny cold; nose is sore; severe sneezing; affects eyes and sinuses; much but mild tearing; symptoms occur after becoming chilled, wet. *Worse:* wetness, cold *Better:* fresh air, head wrapped up warmly	**Cepa**
Mild, watery cold; affects the eyes, much tearing, sharp and burning; edge of eyelid is red; later a thick, slimy mucus gums up the eye. *Worse:* light *Better:* darkness, warmth	**Euphrasia**
Thick, yellow or yellow-greenish stringy nasal discharge; thick drops of mucus; crusts develop; pressure at the base of the nose; spreads to the sinuses. *Worse:* early morning from 3 A.M. on, cold *Better:* warm steam (humidifier), warm weather, fresh air	**Kali bichromicum D12**
Runny nose but hardly any sneezing; headaches; exhausted; tired. *Better:* fresh air NOTE: Particularly effective for a nonspecific beginning of a cold. If nose is stopped-up, use D6.	**Luffa operaculata D12**

KEY SYMPTOMS	REMEDY
Mild, watery cold, particularly during the day; in the evening and during the night, nose is stopped up and dry; nosebleed; extreme sneezing when exposed to cold air; nose itches because of being too often exposed to draft. *Worse:* in the evening, warm rooms *Better:* mild, fresh air	**Nux vomica D12**
Thick yellow or yellow-greenish slimy mucus, mild; often starts on the right side; frequent changes between runny and stuffy nose; bad mood; complains constantly; whines; is restless. *Better:* receiving sympathy, fresh air	**Pulsatilla D12**
Heavy, watery cold; later, thick; severe sneezing; stuffed nose, alternates between the left and right side; nose and eyes are burning; forehead aches; pressure at base of nose. *Worse:* cold air, outside, fragrance from flowers *Better:* warm air, warm drinks	**Sabadilla**
Dry cold with constant itching, develops only slowly; loses sense of smell; inside the nose hard crusts form that bleed when removed; cold spreads easily to the sinuses; oppressive headache, then thick slimy mucus. *Worse:* cold, lying down *Better:* warmth (particularly around the head), moving outside in fresh air	**Silicea D12**

SINUS INFECTION

Bacteria and viruses cause infections of the sinuses, and this can affect both sides of the nose and the upper jawbone (where there is a sinus cavity) as well as above the base of the nose at the forehead and at the temples (the sphenoid bone). A sinus infection is often the result of a cold (see under that topic) and can be a chronic condition. In the case of a serious acute situation accompanied by severe pain, high fever (102° F/39° C), and dizziness, always consult with your physician immediately.

KEY SYMPTOMS	REMEDY
Infection starts quickly with pounding pain in the forehead or sinus cavities; extremely sensitive to vibrations, even talking is too much; face is feverishly hot, bright to dark red; tendency to perspire. *Worse:* nights, cold	**Belladonna D6***
Sinus infection with extreme headaches in the area of the forehead and pressure around the base of the nose; thick, foul-smelling mucus drip into the throat; bad taste in the mouth and throat; would like to rinse the mouth constantly; mouth and throat are dry. *Worse:* nights, dampness, warmth (under the covers) *Better:* fresh air, quiet, cold	**Cinnabaris D12**
Widespread sinus infection with a cough that sets in rather quickly; stabbing, deep-seated headaches in the forehead above the eyes; excess mucus drip into the throat, causing spasm-like coughing spells, particularly during the night; very sensitive to cold air—breathes through a cloth; in bed pulls covers over the head. *Worse:* cold, outdoors *Better:* warm rooms	**Corallium rubrum D6**

*One dose every 30 minutes, but only for 2 hours.

KEY SYMPTOMS	REMEDY

As an aftermath of a cold or being exposed to draft; yellowish-green mucus drips from the nose; first is runny, then is thick and foul-smelling; nostrils are sore, later crusted; pain in the forehead and jaws as if pounded by a nail.
Worse: nights, in the morning, cold draft
Better: warm steam (steam bath), head wrapped up

Hepar sulfuris D4 or D6

As an aftermath of a cold with a burning, runny nose; headaches are one-sided, on the side of the infection; thick, yellowish postnasal drip; pain in scalp and neck muscles.
Worse: nights, warmth, motion
Better: fresh air

Hydrastis D6

Quick progression from having liquid discharge with a feeling of dryness and pressure at the base of the nose to thick, slippery, stringy discharge; builds difficult-to-dislodge crusts; pinpoint pain radiates into the forehead.
Worse: pressure; cold
Better: warm steam (steam bath), warm weather

Kali bichromicum D12

Painful, one- or two-sided sinus infection with severe pain over one or both eyes and at the base of the nose; in the beginning, profuse, burning, acid-like discharge from the nose; later, nose is stuffed; has heavy sneezing fits with tears; swollen eye lids.

Kali jodatum D12

Sinus infection, during the day with migraine headaches; watery discharge or blocked nasal passages; extremely thirsty.

Natrum chloratum D12

HAY FEVER (ALLERGIES)

Hay fever is a cold-like, allergic reaction to plant pollen and other irritants, such as animal hair and house dust. It often coincides with a particular season. Symptoms may spread to the eyes, throat, and bronchial system. The most successful treatment for allergies is a constitutional therapy performed by an experienced physician. IMPORTANT: Do not attempt self-treatment, if you have just gone through a constitutional therapy; rather, let your physician treat you. Also, seek medical treatment in cases of allergic asthma. In addition to the remedies listed under a cold (*Arsenicum album*, *Arum triphyllum*, *Cepa*, *Euphrasia*, *Nux vomica*, and *Sabadilla*), the following remedies have been shown to work well for allergies in their acute phases.

KEY SYMPTOMS	REMEDY
Hay fever in the spring; runny nose with sore nostrils; constant sneezing; blockages; tendency toward asthma. *Worse:* dampness, cold, humid weather, evenings, nights, midnight	**Aralia racemosa**
An extremely watery, runny nose; nostrils and upper lip sore and burning; itchy nose; severe sneezing. *Worse:* warm rooms, very cold air	**Arsenicum jodatum D12**
Severely runny nose with a watery, sharp, hot, or thick yellow discharge; tip of nose is red; severe sneezing; eyes burning and tearing. *Worse:* warm rooms *Better:* fresh air, outdoors	**Kali jodatum D12**
Severely runny nose; nose is sore and burning; severe sneezing; pressure to the base of the nose; unable to smell anything; eyes and throat burning and sore. *Worse:* some fragrances/smells	**Sanguinara canadensis**

CHAPTER 4

EARS, EYES, MOUTH, AND TEETH

EARACHES

The causes of earaches range all the way from slight irritation due to exposure to cold wind to severe bacterial infections of the middle ear with a pus-like discharge (*Otitis media*). Earaches often come in combination with a viral infection or in the aftermath of childhood diseases, like scarlet fever and measles (see also under these terms). Toothaches, particularly those occuring during teething, can also affect the ears. Earaches should only be treated in the very first stage, and then by only an experienced lay person. See your physician if there is no improvement after the first 24 hours. In the case of a rapidly rising temperature, a high temperature (102° F/39° C), severe pain, discharge, or loss of hearing, see your physician immediately.

IMPORTANT: Some remedies that have been proven successful for colds and flus treated at home must only be used for earaches by an experienced homeopath. This holds true particularly for low-potency dosages—up to D4—of *Pulsatilla*, *Hepar sulfuris*, *Sulfur*, and *Lycopodium*.

KEY SYMPTOMS	REMEDY
Very severe onset, usually around midnight; caused by dry, cold wind, often East winds or a draft while driving a car; children, in particular, will whimper or often scream outright for pain; very fearful, anxious, and restless; extremely sensitive to noise; feeling as if water is in the ear; ears are hot and red; shivers; fever increases rapidly; skin is hot and dry; extremely thirsty. *Worse:* after midnight, cold wind, warm rooms, motion *Better:* quiet	**Aconitum D12*/****
Sudden onset; pounding, hammering, or pulsating earaches; pain comes in waves; fever; skin is hot and sweaty. *Worse:* cold, vibrations (even of talking) *Better:* rest/quiet, head elevated	**Belladonna D6***

*One dose every 30 minutes, but for no more than 2 hours.
**If experienced, use l to 2 C30.

KEY SYMPTOMS	REMEDY

Severe, wave-like, stabbing pain in the ears; ears seem to be blocked, sore; ringing in the ears; cheek on the affected side is flushed; particularly for children when teething; very moody and overly sensitive; children throw their toys around in a rage; they want to be carried all the time.
Worse: before midnight, warmth
Better: when shown sympathy, after an outbreak of perspiration, cold drinks

Chamomilla D12

Sudden onset; stabbing pain, also humming in the ears; caused by having gotten chilled due to damp/wet cold weather; change in the weather; often in the fall; tendency to getting colds; low fever.
Worse: nights, cold, wetness
Better: warmth

Dulcamara

Slow onset; pounding or pulsating pain; often caused by viral infection; fever rises only slowly; complexion changes between red and pale.
Worse: in the evening, nights, cold, wet/damp
Better: cold compresses, slow movements

Ferrum phosphoricum D12

Outer ear swollen and red; in the beginning little pain; is hard of hearing; has a feeling as though the ear is plugged up; not thirsty.
Worse: nights
Better: giving sympathy; cold compresses

Pulsatilla D12

NOTE: In cases of frequently recurring ear infections, a constitutional therapy is highly recommended.

EYE STRAIN

The main symptoms of eye strain are increases in tearing, itching, burning, as well as a temporary decrease in vision, particularly at night. Typical causes are computer work in poor light and too little sleep. Make sure that your screen is properly adjusted ergonomically and that you take the necessary breaks and have proper lighting. With increasing age, people need more light. ATTENTION: The following remedies are only to be taken orally. Never apply drops or undiluted tinctures into the eyes. It could cause burning!

KEY SYMPTOMS	REMEDY
Burning pain; increased tearing; forced to blink constantly; letters become blurred; dull headaches; caused by exhaustion or getting a cold. *Worse:* light, wind *Better:* darkness, sleep, rest, warmth	**Euphrasia**
Eyes are red and hot; pressure in the eye socket; headaches; change from far to near vision is difficult; temporarily diminished vision; main reason for strain is close work (reading, sewing, computer), but also from too much TV viewing).	**Ruta graveolens**

NOTE: A sudden loss of vision may also be caused by general exhaustion due to overwork, anemia, severe illness, or pregnancy or having given birth. Seek advice from an experienced physician or homeopath.

STIES

A sty is an infection on the edge of the eyelid or inside the eyelid due to pus-producing bacteria. It often occurs in combination with conjunctivitis and inflammation of the eyelids (see under that topic). Sties can get frightfully large, but in most cases they are harmless. In cases where there is pain or no improvement within four or five days of self-treatment, see your physician.

KEY SYMPTOMS	REMEDY
Eyelids are dry, red, swollen, or cracked; can't tolerate artificial light. Especially for restless, indecisive, and choleric people.	**Graphites**
Eyelids are gummed up, itchy, and burn; the person tries to avoid light; has spasms in the eyelids; the discharge causes sores; particularly in cases of repressed anger and frustrations.	**Staphysagria**
Frequently recurring sties, particularly on the upper lid; thick yellow pus.	**Pulsatilla D12**

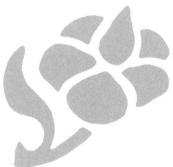

CONJUNCTIVITIS AND INFLAMMATION OF THE EYELIDS

An infection of the conjunctiva and the eyelids often follows a cold or a viral infection. If no improvement is noticed after two to three days, see your physician. If there is a high fever (102° F/39° C), see your physician immediately.

To repeat, the following remedies are always to be taken orally; never use tinctures or undiluted drops directly in the eye. There is danger of burning! Use only those eye drops prescribed by your physician. Also, eye infections are highly infectious; wash hands after having had contact with the infected eye; use wash cloth and towels only once (paper towels are best), and change bed linen every day.

KEY SYMPTOMS	REMEDY
Eyes are hot, dry, and inflamed; severe and burning pain comes on with a vengeance; feels as if sand has got in the eyes; eyelids are swollen; these symptoms are characteristic of beginning stage; is caused by dry/cold wind (east wind) or a draft while driving a car. *Worse:* touch, motion *Better:* quiet/rest	**Aconitum D12*/****
Conjunctiva bright red; tears are hot; stabbing, burning pain as if the eyes are full of sand; eyelids are swollen and glassy. *Worse:* warmth (compresses) *Better:* cold (compresses)	**Apis mellifica**

*One dose every 30 minutes, but for no more than 2 hours.
**If experienced, use 1 to 2 C30.

KEY SYMPTOMS	REMEDY
Sudden onset; conjunctiva red, dry, glassy; burning or stabbing pain; highly sensitive to light; pounding or pulsating headaches; reason often is because of working by strong, glaring light, also can be caused by snow blindness and virus infection; very restless; highly overstimulated or numb; these symptoms are typical for the beginning stages. *Worse:* light, motion *Better:* darkness, quiet/rest	**Belladonna D6***
Conjunctiva and eyelids are inflamed, red, or watery; severe tearing; burning pain but tears are mild; often combined with a severe cold; has headaches in warm rooms. *Worse:* warmth (including compresses) *Better:* coolness, fresh air, outdoors	**Cepa**
Conjunctiva and eyelids are red with burning pain; severe tearing, burning, and hot eyes; eyelids are swollen, sore, and gummed up; has to blink constantly; has dull headaches. *Worse:* light, warmth, winds, in the evening *Better:* darkness, sleep	**Euphrasia**
Itching, burning pain; lots of slimy, thick, mild, yellow discharge; discharge is "swimming" in lots of tears; tendency for developing a sty; cause is usually a cold and/or exposure to draft; is moody; whines. *Worse:* warmth *Better:* fresh air, sympathy, attention	**Pulsatilla D12**

*One dose every 30 minutes, but never exceed 2 hours.

EYE INJURIES

Eye injuries are usually sustained during athletic activities and garden work, from being hit by a ball or poked by a branch or twig. As a matter of course, see an eye specialist when the eye has been injured, even if the injury seems to be minor. Only such a person can judge if the eye indeed has remained intact. The following remedies may be used in addition to the therapy prescribed by the eye specialist and may support the healing process. They are to be used orally only!

KEY SYMPTOMS	REMEDY
Eye feels cold and is bloodshot; injury is dot-shaped, and caused by a blunt object (typical for an injury by a twig or branch). *Worse:* warmth *Better:* cold (compresses)	**Ledum D6**
The remedy is the main medication when there has been a dull bruise caused by a ball or a punch; painful hematoma in and around the eye (black eye).	**Symphytum D6**

NOTE: First-aid remedies until the person gets to the eye specialist: every 15 minutes *Ledum* D6 or *Symphytum* D6.

GINGIVITIS

Gingivitis is an infection of the gums, usually resulting from small injuries: for example, a bite that doesn't line up properly and burns from hot food or hot liquids. It can also occur during a flu and during pregnancy, often spreading throughout the mouth cavity. In case of severe complaints, bluish-red or blue discoloration, high fever (102° F/39° C), ulcers, tearing, or pus, see your physician or dentist immediately.

KEY SYMPTOMS	REMEDY
Gums are pale to light red, glassy, and swollen; hot stabbing pain; often infection has spread throughout the mouth cavity. *Worse:* warm drinks *Better:* cold drinks	**Apis mellifica**
Sudden onset; bright red swelling; burning, stabbing, throbbing pain; extreme sense of dryness; is drinking cold water in smalls sips, even though the pain gets worse in the process; tongue often is raspberry red. *Worse:* in the evening, nights, after eating	**Belladonna D6***
Dark red swelling; stabbing pain; usually in an advanced stage; if you see white spots or white blisters, consult your physician immediately.	**Phytolacca**

NOTE: Frequently reappearing infections are either due to mechanical problems, poorly fitting dentures, or the sharp edges or corners on one or more teeth. But they can also be the result of poor dental hygiene or of a general weakness of the body's defense mechanism. For those reasons, first check with your dentist and then have an experienced homeopath prescribe a constitutional therapy.

*One dose every 30 minutes, but never exceed 2 hours.

ACUTE TOOTHACHES

A sudden toothache is a sign of a cavity and/or a bacterial infection around a tooth. See your dentist immediately. The following remedies are only meant to make the waiting time more bearable.

KEY SYMPTOMS	REMEDY
Sudden onset; pounding, pulsating, or throbbing pain, often on the right side; head feels hot, is flushed; cheek is swollen. *Worse:* in cold, cold wind, in the evening, nights, after eating *Better:* sitting in semi-upright position	**Belladonna D6***
Stabbing pain; moves from one tooth to another; person is moody; irritated; rejecting; wants to be left alone. *Worse:* nights, brushing teeth, smoking, warmth (food and drink) *Better:* lying down or pressure on the painful side, cold water (rinsing)	**Bryonia**
Unbearable pain; wants to hit head against a wall; pain often on right side; cheek is hot, red, and swollen; gums often burning hot; pain causes perspiration to break out on forehead; often during pregnancy; person is very aggressive, restless, and feels that the situation is unfair. *Worse:* warmth in any form, coffee, in the evening, at night *Better:* apply cold (ice bag), cold drinks	**Chamomilla D12**

*One dose every 30 minutes, but not more than 4 doses.

KEY SYMPTOMS   REMEDY

Stabbing, shooting pain that comes and goes
in short intervals; attacks are unbearable;
crying because of the pain and exhaustion;
anxious and restless.
Worse: warm food, in the evening, nights,
warmth of the bed
Better: ice-cold water (rinsing or ice cubes)

Coffea D12

Highly sensitive, cavity-plagued teeth;
aching pain that often radiates to the ears;
often triggered during a meal; pulsating pain
in the temples; cheeks swollen; gums are
swollen and sensitive to touch; gums tend to
bleed.
Worse: cold, cold drinks, cold air
Better: warmth, pressure (clenching teeth)

Staphysagria

TEETHING PROBLEMS

Main remedy for restless children; they don't
know what they want and are unpleasant;
screaming; raging; have interrupted sleep; often
accompanied by fever and sore bottom.
Better: being carried, riding in a car

Chamomilla D12

Main remedy for restless children; gums
are swollen; head perspires heavily; often
accompanied by diarrhea; eruption of permanent
teeth is delayed.
Worse: cold, cold drinks
Better: rest, quiet

Calcarea carbonica

DISCOMFORT AFTER DENTAL TREATMENT

Letting your dentist treat your "sick" teeth usually removes the worst pain. However, discomfort in the area where treatment has been performed usually lasts for some time afterwards. This pain is usually caused by small injuries of the surrounding gingiva, pressure on the side of the teeth and jaws, and, of course, soreness from the wound after an extraction. If the following remedies do not coincide with the characteristics of the symptoms or don't bring relief within six hours, check the section on Sensitive Teeth or see your dentist.

KEY SYMPTOMS	REMEDY
Dull or aching pain after treatment (fillings, fitting a crown, etc.); injury to gingiva due to removal of tartar; post-operative bleeding; pressure pain or sore spots from new dentures.	**Arnica D12***
Pain and soreness after extraction of a tooth; severe nerve pain. *Worse:* during the night	**Hypericum D6***
Gnawing, stabbing pain after a filling; feels like the pain from a needle; general nausea, particularly after local anesthesia; very sensitive to cold. *Better:* warm drinks, warm compresses.	**Nux vomica D12***

*Depending on severity, 1 dose every 30 to 60 minutes in potency indicated potency, but no more than 5 total.

SENSITIVE TEETH

Sensitive teeth react to contact with food that is warm, cold, sweet, or sour; they also react to movement and touch. It is essential to let your dentist establish a proper diagnosis. If the neck of a root is exposed, the dentist can prescribe a medication that helps to remineralize the affected area.

KEY SYMPTOMS	REMEDY
Very sensitive to dry, cold wind, including draft when driving in a car; pulsating, unbearable pain; tongue and mouth are either numb or burning hot; face is hot and red; often occurs during a cold. *Worse:* dry, cold wind, warm room, in the evening, nights *Better:* quiet/rest, fresh air	**Aconitum D12**
Very sensitive to cold or touch; pain travels from one tooth to another; also suitable for after dental treatment. *Worse:* cold in any form, touch *Better:* warmth in any form, pressure	**Magnesium phosphoricum**
Very sensitive to cold; gnawing or pulling pain; often during a cold but also after mental stress; person is hypochondriacal, moody, and bossy. *Worse:* cold, draft, cold drinks, coffee, in the morning, nights, after eating *Better:* warm drinks	**Nux vomica D12**
Very sensitive to touch; teeth feel as if they are too long; stabbing, gnawing, or pulling pain; pain attacks are unbearable; pain radiates to the ears, alternating between ear and tooth; cheek is swollen; heavy flow of saliva; also good for after a dental treatment. *Worse:* touch, fresh air, extreme temperatures *Better:* rest/quiet, lying down, moderately warm room	**Plantago major**

LOSS OF TEETH
(CAVITIES)

Loosing one's teeth is usually caused by poor dental hygiene and poor nutrition. Also, antibiotics (particularly tetracycline) given to children under the age of 10 years have been known to weaken their teeth. For some people, of course, the poor "quality" of their teeth might also have been inherited. Homeopathic remedies, needless to say, won't fix a cavity; but they can be helpful in protecting healthy teeth from additional damage. Constitutional therapy would be very helpful and is highly recommended, provided it is performed by an experienced homeopath.

Dosage: 3 times daily, one standard dose of D6 for no longer than three months.

KEY SYMPTOMS	REMEDY
Cavities already beginning in early child-hood (in toddlers and children of school age).	**Acidum fluoricum**
Tooth development is slow, but teeth become susceptible to cavities rather quickly.	**Calcarea phosphorica**
Cavities developing after too many sweets, including lemonade; heavy saliva flow.	**Coccinella**
Cavities developing very quickly; teeth are dark and crumbling; gums are spongy, bleeding; foul mouth odor; bitter taste.	**Kreosotum**
Loss of teeth during menopause, particularly due to periodontosis and receding gums; very sensitive labially (at the gum line); cavities along the gum line.	**Thuja**

CHAPTER 5

Skin, Nails, and Hair

BASIC INFORMATION

Problem skin, nails, and hair are usually symptoms that indicate more deep-seated imbalances, not only those of a physical nature but also emotional and mental imbalances. Often, as in the case of skin rashes, the type of symptom a person exhibits can indicate what the underlying causes of the problem might be. Illustrative examples are measles, chicken pox, and scarlet fever. Some complaints, like frequently occurring skin rashes (the so-called wind-induced dermatitis), could well be signs of other problems, such as a disfunctioning liver or an imbalance in the production of perspiration. Similarly, these imbalances could be indicated by hair and nail problems, like extreme hair loss or brittle nails. As we have said: Always look at the total person when choosing a homeopathic remedy.

Of course, some complaints result from local irritation, such as sunburn or corns due to poor footwear. In such cases, treatment with homeopathic remedies is designed to bring relief and support healing of the acute problem. The reason the symptom appeared in the first place must be rectified by the patient. In the examples mentioned, less sun bathing and more comfortable shoes, respectively, would be appropriate actions to take.

Self-treatment for skin, hair, and nail problems ought to be done only after the underlying reasons have been determined. And here, take note of the following: If the problems are caused by some basic imbalance, it is recommended that after the acute symptoms have been treated, a constitutional therapy be considered by an experienced homeopath. This even holds true for a seemingly isolated event like an eczema that has been caused by nickel-containing fashion jewelry.

In the following instances it is essential to seek medical advice immediately (if necessary, even at an emergency facility):

- as soon as a localized infection seems to be either spreading, reaching deeper layers of the tissue, in case of high fever (102° F/39° C), or there is severe pain
- when skin rashes appear immediately after having taken medication (for instance, antibiotics). If existing complaints are accompanied by additional problems, like headaches or breathing difficulty, immediately or shortly after having taken medication, go to an emergency room at once.

NOTE: For injuries to the skin, see Chapter 11.

ABSCESSES

An abscess is a festering bacterial infection. One type affects individual sebaceous glands and hair roots, and these are called boils; the other type affects a larger area, involving several glands and hair roots, and this is termed a carbuncle. Self-treatment is recommended only by an experienced lay person. A carbuncle must always be treated by a physician. Seek medical advice immediately if infections and inflammations seem to get worse (particularly around the head) and if the pain increases.

KEY SYMPTOMS	REMEDY
Early stages of pustule: skin is hot, red, swollen; person has pounding pain.	**Belladonna**
Festering continues even after it has been lanced; pustule is thick and slimy; crusts over easily.	**Calcarea sulfurica**
Pustule is yellowish-green; stabbing, cutting pain; very sensitive to touch. *Worse:* cold	**Hepar sulfuris**
In the early stages:	**C30***
Abscess almost ripe:	**D4****
Lancing a ripe carbuncle.	**Myristica sebifera D6****
Festering won't stop in spite of having been lanced; discharge is thin and foul-smelling; edges of the wound are festering, inflamed, and hard. Particularly for people who are always cold.	**Silicea**

*One to 2 doses. In case of recurring abscesses, do not continue using C30, but seek medical attention immediately.
** 5 times a day, standard dose.
***Every 2 hours, 5 drops dilution.

SKIN BLEMISHES AND ACNE

These problems occur most frequently during puberty. But they are also prevalent where the immune system has been weakened, where a hormonal imbalance in the female monthly cycle exists, and where constipation is a problem. Cosmetics can also be the culprit. Methods of prevention include careful hygiene, low-fat, high-fiber food with plenty of raw vegetables, no sugar, little meat, plenty of fresh air and sun, and exercise.

Dosage: 3 times daily of standard dose D6 or once a day D12; but for no longer than 6 weeks.

KEY SYMPTOMS	REMEDY
Acne; festering, knotted pustules; surrounding area is also knotty; especially in case where problem also with constipation; thick, white layer on the surface of the tongue.	**Antimonium crudum**
Severe acne; hard, brown-colored but painless pustules. Especially in thin, restless people. *Worse:* in the spring	**Arsenicum bromatum**
Symptoms similar to those in *Arsenicum bromatum*, but in slightly plump people with light skin and blond hair. *Better:* on the beach	**Bromum**
Blemished skin due to the use of cosmetics; also after conventional therapy. *Worse:* summer: bathing and swimming	**Bovista**
Oily skin due to the use of cosmetics; skin is limp, pale, damp/cold; face looks pasty; head sweaty during the night. Especially for light-skinned, slow, and lethargic people.	**Calcarea carbonica**
Acne; hard, bluish-brownish knots, also on the back and upper body; severe itch. *Worse:* menstruation	**Kali bromatum**

KEY SYMPTOMS	REMEDY
Oily, shiny, light skin; particularly at the hair line and around the eyes. *Worse:* sun, at the beach	**Natrum chloratum**
Blemishes on forehead due mainly to use of cosmetics; also during bouts of constipation and the misuse of laxatives.	**Nux vomica D12**
Blemished skin caused by eating pork; also in case of delayed and minimal menstruation. *Worse:* during menstruation, fatty foods	**Pulsatilla D12**
Facial skin oily and shiny; many dark black-heads; acne; chills easily but can't stand warmth. *Worse:* during menstruation	**Selenium**
Dark, blotchy, yellowish-pale skin; dark circles under the eye; especially when menstruation is delayed, and when there is total exhaustion.	**Sepia**
Acne; hard pustules; slowly developing pustules. Especially for people who are constantly cold.	**Silicea**
Rough, dry, red skin; looks unhealthy and uncared for; face is covered with pustules and blackheads; washing face is uncomfortable. *Worse:* warmth, water	**Sulfur**
As in *Sulfur*, but especially for acne accompanied by hard pustules.	**Sulfur jodatum**
Blemished skin after immunization and due to the consumption of protein-rich food, particularly animal protein; oily skin.	**Thuja**

DERMATITIS

The most common skin rashes (urticaria) are caused by contact with an irritating plant, such as the nettle weed or poison ivy, but often also caused by a sensitivity to certain foods, some medications, animal hair, and insect bites. Cases of acute stomach and intestinal problems can also cause a rash. In case of high fever (102° F/39° C) or if the overall well-being is severely affected, seek medical advice. In cases of frequently occurring dermatitis, a constitutional therapy administered by an experienced homeopath is recommended. IMPORTANT: In cases of allergic reaction to medication and insect bites where the symptoms include headaches, nausea, and breathing difficulties, seek medical care immediately.

KEY SYMPTOMS	REMEDY
A measles-like rash in combination with an upset stomach, particularly after meat consumption; nausea and vomiting that does not bring relief; tongue is covered with a white thick layer.	**Antimonium crudum**
Burning, stabbing pain with itching; skin is pale red to pale blue. *Worse:* touch, warmth, perspiring, a change in the weather *Better:* coolness, cold	**Apis mellifica**
Rash due to the consumption of spoiled protein (meat, fish); intense, burning pain; restless during the night. *Worse:* scratching *Better:* hot compresses; itching is sometimes also relieved with cold compresses	**Arsenicum D12**
Intolerance to milk; development of lumps. *Better:* cool air	**Calcarea carbonica**

KEY SYMPTOMS	REMEDY

Red, itching blotches after having become
chilled or clothing has become soaked; also
occurs prior to the onset of menstruation;
especially in case of rheumatic joint problems.
 Paradoxical modalities:
  If there is a rash with itching:
 Worse: warmth, motion
 Better: cold air
  If there are joint problems:
 Better: warmth, motion

Dulcamara

Burning pain with itching; skin red; often
after a cold bath. Especially for people
sensitive to cold and wetness who suffer
from rheumatism and gout problems.
Better: warmth and pressure

Formica rufa

Cannot tolerate shellfish. Especially for people
who are introverted and unforgiving.

Natrum chloratum

Cannot tolerate fish; often has an aversion to it;
after an allergic reaction to penicillin. Especially
for people with transparent skin.

Phosphorus

Burning pain; skin is swollen and red;
develops blisters and lumps; often after
having become wet and cold in the spring.
Worse: cold air, sweating

**Rhus
toxicodendron**

Cannot tolerate fish; develops lumps.
Especially for women who experience
difficulty with their menstruation or problems
during menopause.
Worse: cold air

Sepia

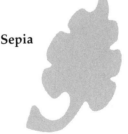

KEY SYMPTOMS	REMEDY
Contact allergies; medication-induced rashes; burning pain; intense itching; bright red blisters. Especially for people with dry, rough, and blemished skin that heals only poorly. *Worse:* scratching, warm bed, water	**Sulfur**
Burning pain; severe itching, "ants crawling" (a feeling as if something is crawling under the skin), tingling heat; also in case of an intolerance to mussels. *Worse:* warmth, physical stress *Better:* coolness, cold	**Urtica urens**

SUN ALLERGIES

This is an allergic reaction that occurs when skin is exposed to too much sun. Usually the skin develops blisters, a rash, or an eczema, with and without itching. It should not to be confused with sunburn. After treatment of the acute complaints, a constitutional therapy by an experienced homeopath is recommended .

KEY SYMPTOMS	REMEDY
Red-colored blisters and pustules; intense itching. *Worse:* warmth (also warm bed)	**Acidum hydrochloricum**
Wounds and knot-like blisters on slightly sweaty skin; intense itching.	**Hypericum**
Rash, similar to a contact dermatitis, herpes, or a gritty eruption; skin is dry, oily, and shiny; also increased production from the sebaceous glands. *Worse:* on the beach	**Natrum chloratum**
Wounds and blisters with dry skin. Especially for blond or reddish-blond people with light, transparent skin.	**Phosphorus**

KEY SYMPTOMS	REMEDY
Eczema similar to a contact rash; small knotty blisters (heat blisters), particularly at the back of the neck, shoulder, arms, and legs; sometimes moist; sometimes tendency to have heat-induced edema in the legs.	Pulsatilla D12

WARTS

Warts are skin colored, yellow, or grayish-brown and are sometimes callused, flat, or elevated on the skin. Caused by a viral infection, they can be prevented by avoiding skin contact with people who have them. If warts that have been present for some time begin to bleed, become wet, change appearance (in color and/or size), or if new, dark warts appear, see your physician immediately in order to eliminate the possibility of skin cancer. Ask your homeopath for a tincture for external application.

KEY SYMPTOMS	REMEDY
Wide, hard; particularly on fingers and the sole of feet with callus.	Antimonium crudum
Hard, callous; jagged; often been present for a long time; often on fingers, hands, soles of the feet; sometimes also stemmed in the face, nose, eyelid; surface very rough and easily injured, then painful.	Causticum
Especially in people with a very transparent skin; also for young girls during puberty and people who get exhausted quickly.	Ferrum picricum
Main remedy for soft, furrowed, yellowish brown, and stemmed warts on hands, fingers, face, neck, and back.	Thuja

IRRITATED SKIN

Irrtitation occurs in creases of the skin, like the armpit, behind the knee, under the breasts, and in the area of the buttocks. Usually sore skin is caused by an increase in perspiration and friction. This condition is especially prevalent in people with weight problems. If a skin fungus is suspected, see your physician.

KEY SYMPTOMS	REMEDY
Slight soreness; one-time or rare occurrence caused by tight or wrong clothing; also can be caused by other unfamiliar physical stress.	**Calendula powder**
Skin is bright red with throbbing pain; especially when due to increased perspiration, physical stress, or illness accompanied by fever.	**Belladonna**
Extreme perspiration; nightly sweat around the head; skin damp, cold, loose, and pale. Especially for slow-developing children and lethargic people.	**Calcarea carbonica**
Increased perspiration with hot flashes during menopause.	**Sanguinara**
Extreme perspiration with hot flashes; skin is dry, hard, and red; has aversion to wate. Especially for children and active, self-absorbed people. *Worse:* warmth, in the spring, humid weather	**Sulfur**

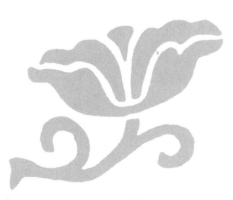

DIAPER RASH

Skin rashes in babies and children in the area that is covered by diapers occur often after changes in feeding habits—when the mother goes from nursing to giving supplemental feedings—or as the result of the ingestion of unfamiliar, acid-containing food (oranges, tomatoes). A diaper rash can also be caused by a sensitivity to sugar. IMPORTANT: Keep the infant or child's bottom as dry as possible (change diapers often or use no diapers at all and use the warm setting of a hair dryer to dry the skin). If a yeast/fungus infection (*Candida albicans*) should set in (recognizable by watery blisters that are close together), or if a bladder infection is suspected, seek medical advice immediately.

KEY SYMPTOMS	REMEDY
Urine is foul-smelling, extremely sour; skin is red and itches; the child wants to be comforted and held/carried; often accompanied by diarrhea from unfamiliar or sour food.	Acidum benzoicum
Rash is particularly prevalent during teething; the child is very moody; whining; throws temper tantrums; wants to be carried constantly.	Chamomilla D12
Pale to light red pustules, similar to chicken pox; skin is swollen; extremely itchy; hot.	Rhus toxicodendron

HAIR LOSS

Hair loss is not unusual, often occurring after a long illnesses, hormonal changes after pregnancy/birth, during menopause, because of poor nutrition. It can also be due to emotional stress after difficult events. If the hair is lost in round patches or occurs after having taken conventional medication or radiation therapy, always seek the advice of an experienced homeopath. If a thyroid problem is suspected at all, see your physician.

Dosage: once a day, 1 standard dose of D12 for a maximum of 6 weeks.

KEY SYMPTOMS	REMEDY
Hair loss due to emotional reasons; also hair turning gray spontaneously; especially after worry, including lovesickness; does not care, is lethargic; lacks concentration.	**Acidum phosphoricum**
Scalp is itchy, often accompanied by dandruff; has a burning sensation during the night; can't stand combing; extremely exhausted, anxious, restless; especially after an illness.	**Arsenicum album**
Hair loss after having given birth; scalp extremely itchy, which forces constant scratching.	**Calcarea carbonica**
Head sweaty during the night. Especially prevalent in people with weight problems and light, pasty-looking facial skin.	
Hair loss due to emotional stress; especially after worries; also after too much mental activity; especially during preparations for exams.	**Kali phosphoricum**
Hair loss during pregnancy. Especially for women whose mental and emotional state has changed considerably during pregnancy.	**Lachesis**

KEY SYMPTOMS	REMEDY
Hair loss after having given birth; also hair loss due to premature aging with distinct wrinkles across the forehead; premature graying.	**Lycopodium**
Hair loss after having given birth, prolonged nursing; during menopause; especially at the hairline and receding hairline; extremely exhausted; weight loss from "the top on down."	**Natrum chloratum**
Hair coming out in patches, leaves bare spots; extremely exhausted, tired. Especially for people with fine hair when scalp is visible after an illness, and in cases of premature aging.	**Phosphorus**
Hair loss after having given birth; during menopause; skin is pale yellow with dark circles under the eyes; a feeling as if the uterus is sagging; varicose veins; completely exhausted; nervous; sad.	**Sepia**
Sensitive scalp; constantly cold but can tolerate only a very light, soft hat; tendency toward cold sweaty feet and head—rest of the body otherwise dry; often blotchy nails. Especially in young people after recovering from an illness.	**Silicea**
Hair loss due to emotional stress; heavy dandruff; hair loss is severe and quick; especially after having been hurt; has angry reactions or tends to brood and withdraw.	**Staphysagria**
Thallium is the main remedy for hair loss after an acute illness accompanied by severe exhaustion. IMPORTANT: The illness must have been of a general kind, such as a severe infection with high fever.	**Thallium**

CORNS AND CALLUSES

Corns and calluses are usually the result of misaligned bones in the feet or inappropriate shoes. These would be shoes that are either the wrong kind, are too tight, have heels that are too high, or don't have proper support built into them. If complaints occur frequently, see a podiatrist. Let a homeopath prescribe a tincture to apply to the corns.

KEY SYMPTOMS	REMEDY
Hard, crusty calluses, particularly on the heels; often deep fissures; extreme pain, stabbing, burning; especially where there are also digestive problems.	**Antimonium crudum**
Causticum is the main remedy for corns; for use in case of burning, heavy pain; especially if there is presence of rheumatism in the legs. *Better:* warmth (warm bed)	**Causticum**
Infected corn with extreme, heavy, throbbing, searing, stabbing pain; often one foot is cold, the other warm; especially in the presence of foul-smelling, sticky perspiration coming from underarms and feet.	**Lycopodium**
During changes in the weather; burning, stabbing, piercing pain; especially in cases where there are gout problems in toes and fingers. *Worse:* damp weather, weather changes, feet hanging down	**Ranunculus sceleratus**
Corns very painful; frequently inflamed. Especially for women who have varicose veins.	**Sepia**
Heavy buildup of calluses covering the soles of the feet; dull, burning pain; corns are sore with stabbing pain; feet are ice-cold; strong, foul-smelling foot perspiration; cold most of the time.	**Silicea**

BRITTLE NAILS

Brittle nails are usually due to a mineral deficiency and inadequate nutrition. This condition also often occurs after a serious illness and emotional stress. In cases where there are deep tears and total loss of the nails, a diseased nailbed, and a suspicion of a fungus infection, see your physician. Dosage: one standard dose of D12 once a day over a maximum of 6 weeks.

KEY SYMPTOMS	REMEDY
Nails are brittle, deformed, with vertical ridges; nails grow very fast; has a sense that a splinter might be lodged under the nail. *Worse:* in the summer	**Acidum hydrochoricum**
Nails peeling in layers; brittle, thick, deformed; have small white spots; especially in conjunction with dry skin/mucous membranes.	**Alumina**
Nails peeling in large layers; thick; deep vertical ridges/tears; severe buildup of calluses.	**Antimonium crudum**
Slow physical development in children; heavy perspiration around the head during the night; sweaty/cold hands and feet; moves feet out from under the covers.	**Calcarea carbonica**
Nails peeling in layers; brittle, thick, deformed; often ingrown toenails; especially in conjunction with weight problems and constipation.	**Graphites**
Nails split easily; thickened, deformed; vertical ridges; ridges have white spots. Especially in people who are constantly cold, including children.	**Silicea**
Nails are very soft, brittle; split easily; peeling off in layers; have indentations, ridges; have wave-like horizontal ridges; often in conjunction with ingrown toenails.	**Thuja**

INJURED NAILS

KEY SYMPTOMS	REMEDY
Injuries under the nail due to a splinter or needle; pain is reduced when cold compresses are applied.	Ledum
Black-and-blue discoloration (hematoma) under the nail due to injury; severe pain.	Arnica D12
Shooting, aching pain due to an injury to the tip of the finger without a hematoma present.	Hypericum

NAIL BITING

A sign of repressed emotion, like anger or aggression, nail biting is most frequently found in children but can also occur among adults. Try to determine the cause. If the condition is persistent, seek advice from an experienced homeopath. Dosage: one standard dose D12 once a day for a maximum of 4 weeks.

KEY SYMPTOMS	REMEDY
Nervous irritation; itching under the nails, particularly in the area close to the fingertip; biting is the only relief. Prevalent especially in people who are timid, anxious, and shy.	Ammonium bromatum
Chews nails until they bleed; pulls and scratches nose or lips until the skin comes off in patches. Especially in people who are nervous, restless, and depressed.	Arum triphyllum
Chews and sucks on the tip of the fingers until the bed of the nail is cracked. Especially in children who always look unwashed and unkempt.	Sulfur

CHAPTER 6

DIGESTIVE PROBLEMS

STOMACH AND INTESTINAL UPSET

An upset stomach is usually caused by eating spoiled food, but can also be the result of heavy, unfamiliar meals eaten in a rush, or from taking in too much alcohol and/or nicotine. Discomfort usually starts a few hours after the meal. IMPORTANT: When complaints are severe, and if food poisoning is suspected, see your physician immediately. Babies and small children must be treated by a physician.

KEY SYMPTOMS	REMEDY
Weak stomach; thick, white coating on the tongue; burping tastes of undigested food; vomiting does not bring relief; intolerance to sour food, baked goods, pork, black tea, nicotine, and alcohol.	**Antimonium crudum**
Severe diarrhea/vomiting with shivers; very weak; restless; fear; burning pain in the stomach; extremely thirsty; drinking water in small sips; especially useful in the early stages of food poisoning, after eating ice cream, vinegar, or cucumbers. *Worse:* during the night, midday, cold drinks, cold *Better:* warmth (except around the head)	**Arsenicum album D12**
Food sits in the stomach like a rock; lips, mouth, and tongue are dry; extreme thirst for cold water; nausea, vomiting; also, a summer cold due to damp cold weather. *Worse:* motion, no matter how slight	**Bryonia**
Distended stomach, often in combination with trouble breathing; cramp-like, sharp stomach pain after spoiled food; burping; foul-smelling diarrhea; very weak; pale complexion with cold sweat; also in case of meat-, fat-, milk-intolerance and having eaten too many different things. *Better:* fanning fresh air	**Carbo vegetabilis**

KEY SYMPTOMS	REMEDY
Constantly feeling sick; nausea; vomiting brings no relief; afterwards very weak; cold sweat; tongue is clear; increased saliva flow; not very thirsty; diarrhea looks like spinach; migraine-like headaches with dizziness; especially after difficult-to-digest, fatty food. *Worse:* motion, extreme temperatures	Ipecacuanha
Hangover after too much beer; a dirty-yellow coating of the tongue; feeling bloated; burning stomach pain. *Better:* eating bread	**Kali bichromicum**
Main remedy for stomach problems due to hastily eaten, sumptuous, heavy, highly spiced or unfamiliar food; alcohol and nicotine misuse; also in cases of a flu that has settled in the stomach; food sits in the stomach like a stone; a whitish-yellow coating of the tongue, sour burping, bitter; not very thirsty. *Better:* warmth	Nux vomica
Food sits in the stomach like a stone, particularly after fatty, sweet and sour foods, pork, ice cream, and eating too many different types of food; burping tastes rancid; dirty-white coating of the tongue; mouth is dry but patient is not thirsty; nausea; vomits undigested food and warm drinks. *Better:* cool fresh air	**Pulsatilla D12**
Extreme, watery vomiting diarrhea and nausea; cramp-like abdominal pain after eating spoiled food; a tendency to collapse; body is ice-cold; cold sweat on the forehead; pale, gaunt complexion; mouth dry; feeling of thirst and hunger—everything is vomited up again immediately. *Worse:* motion, no matter how slight	**Veratrum album**

STOMACH AND INTESTINAL FLU

This flu, which is often part of a systemic infection and usually is accompanied by a fever, frequently appears at specific times of the year and has a tendency to afflict the population at large. It can also be the result of a cold caused by consuming very cold foods, particularly cold drinks and ice cream. In cases of high fever (102° F/39° C) and severely reduced overall well-being combined with a weak circulatory system, seek medical attention immediately.

In addition to the remedies listed under Stomach and Intestinal Upset (*Arsenicum album, Bryonia, Nux vomica,* and *Pulsatilla*), the following remedies have also been shown to be effective.

KEY SYMPTOMS	REMEDY
Diarrhea with slightly elevated temperature; feeling as if the colon is about to tear apart; nausea, sour burping; vomiting; tongue coated in the center; bad breath; foul-smelling sweat. *Worse:* fat *Better:* rest/quiet, warmth	**Acidum nitricum**
Acute diarrhea, foul-smelling; gas odorless; stabbing abdomen pain; feeling as if the skin is being pierced by icicles; especially when chilled; also after excitement; exertion.	**Agarius**
Watery summer diarrhea; shows undigested food; cramp-like abdomenal pain with flatulence; can't handle sour foods. Especially for people with weak stomachs who like to eat too much. *Worse:* hot weather, cool bath	**Antimonium crudum**
Diarrhea which shows undigested food; has a fever and severe abdomenal aches; severe burping; flatulence but passing gas brings no relief; fever varies; bitter taste in the mouth. *Worse:* hot weather, milk, fruit *Better:* pressure, bending over	**Colocynthis**

KEY SYMPTOMS	REMEDY
Diarrhea is thick and slimy and occurs with fever; slow onset with abdomenal pain; body ice-cold but person is still thirsty for something cold. Especially for those catching cold in late summer due to having become chilled or wet. *Better:* warmth	**Dulcamara**
Watery diarrhea in the morning, foul-smelling, but without pain; also summer diarrhea; very exhausted; yellow coating of the tongue; teeth leave indentation on the tongue; elimination with abdominal pain immediately after eating; thirsty for something cold. *Better:* bending over, warmth (body compress)	**Podophyllum**

NERVOUS STOMACH AND INTESTINAL PROBLEMS

These problems are usually the result of stress and emotional burdens that have "hit" the stomach. The main symptoms are heartburn, stomach pain, nausea, vomiting, and diarrhea. If these problems occur frequently or have existed for some time, and if ulcers in the stomach or small intestines are suspected, see your physician immediately.

KEY SYMPTOMS	REMEDY
Heavy, aching stomach pain; stops when eating; ravenous appetite; a sense as if a plug is obstructing the rectum and unable to pass stool; mental stress, often occurs before a test. *Better:* eating, lying down, warmth	**Anacardium**
Nausea, cramp-like stomach pain; diarrhea; before important events; after worry. Especially for anxious people who are always in a hurry. *Worse:* eating, warmth, confined space, tight clothes *Better:* fresh air, cold	**Argentum nitricum**

KEY SYMPTOMS	REMEDY
Burning stomach pain; strong urge to drink cold water; swallows the water in small amounts. Eespecially for anxious and restless people who have difficulty being by themselves. *Worse:* in the evening, at night, in darkness	**Arsenicum album D12**
Nausea after eating; food sits in the stomach like a rock; drinks a great amount of cold water. Especially for irritated people who have a temper and can't tolerate opposition. *Worse:* touch, motion, warm rooms *Better:* pressure, warm stomach compress, rest/quiet	**Bryonia**
Nausea with flatulence and colic-like pain; foul-smelling diarrhea that is slimy or "like spinach." Especially for highly irritated or angry people who overreact; also for children during teething.	**Chamomilla D12**
Stomach cramps with diarrhea after anger or rage. Especially for impatient people who show their emotions openly. *Better:* warmth, bending over, pressure	**Colocynthis**
Stomach pain; feeling that stomach is empty; hungry with nausea after distress or sadness. Especially for depressed, introverted people who sigh and cry frequently. *Worse:* light food, sympathy *Better:* heavy food, being alone	**Ignatia**
Heartburn; stabbing, heavy stomach pain; flatulence; nausea; vomiting; diarrhea as well as constipation. Especially for people who bury themselves in old troubles. *Worse:* heat, cold, sympathy	**Natrum chloratum**

KEY SYMPTOMS	REMEDY
Food sits in the stomach like a rock; nausea; heartburn; feeling stuffed; flatulence; diarrhea or constipation; has urge to burp but can't. Especially for ambitious people.	**Nux vomica D12**
Nausea; vomiting; diarrhea after excitement. Especially for people with very a sensitive "antenna."	**Phosphorus**
Nausea; cramp-like heavy stomach pain after being disappointed or hurt. Especially for people who are irritable and moody but accommodating.	**Pulsatilla D12**
Sharp stomach pain; foul-smelling flatulence; diarrhea after being insulted or upset. Especially for people who are introverted but explode suddenly.	**Staphysagria**

HEARTBURN

Heartburn occurs when stomach fluids rise up into the esophagus, particularly when lying down after eating or after drinking coffee, alcohol, or fruit juices. Before starting self-treatment, always check with your physician so as to eliminate possibly serious stomach illnesses. IMPORTANT: Those who have already been treated with conventional remedies (antacid medication) or have taken such remedies on their own ought to check with an experienced homeopath before using any homeopathic remedies.

KEY SYMPTOMS	REMEDY
Strong, sour burping; heartburn; vomiting; the whole person smells sour; particularly prevalent in children and those with a sense of coldness and weakness in the stomach. Especially for people who are exhausted; also people who feel weak after the misuse of alcohol. *Worse:* cold water *Better:* alcohol	**Acidum sulfuricum**
Burning sensation in stomach and esophagus; distinct feeling of cold in the stomach; especially after too much nicotine and/or alcohol. *Worse:* after eating, after drinking	**Capsicum**
Foul-tasting, burning burping; cramp-like burning stomach pain with distended upper abdomen; cannot tolerate meat, fatty foods, or milk; also when too many different kinds of food have been eaten at one time.	**Carbo vegetabilis**
Sour burping, tastes of undigested food; particularly after milk, tea, fruit; pressure and a feeling of "emptiness" in the stomach; has urge for something sour, sweet, for strong alcohol, coffee, and cold water. *Worse:* after eating, touch *Better:* pressure	**China**

KEY SYMPTOMS	REMEDY
Burning sensation in the stomach and esophagus; increases flow of saliva; nausea, sour burping; vomiting of water and sour stomach content is irritating throat, mouth, and tongue; often in combination with migraine headache. *Worse:* usually on days off work	**Iris**
Everything is sour: burping, vomit, and stool; has intolerance to fat, milk, vinegar, sour fruit, sweets, cold drinks, and cold meals; yellow, creamy coating on the tongue and palate. Especially for people who are exhausted and suffer from rheumatic illnesses or gout.	**Natrum phosphoricum**
Main remedy for heartburn that is due to eating heavy, sumptuous, highly spiced or unfamiliar food; misuse of nicotine and/or alcohol; burping tastes sour and bitter; heavy feeling in the stomach. Especially for people who are ambitious, choleric, and pedantic. *Worse:* after the meal *Better:* warmth, rest/quiet	**Nux vomica D12**
Stomach pain with burning heartburn; foul taste in the mouth; can't handle heavy meals, especially pork fat and milk; also after eating too many different foods at one sitting. *Worse:* rest, warmth *Better:* fresh air, motion	**Pulsatilla D12**
Burning pain in the upper part of the abdomen; sour-tasting burping and vomit that makes teeth feel dull; often comes in combination with headaches in forehead or temples; dizziness; cannot tolerate fatty foods or fresh bread. *Worse:* during the night *Better:* after eating	**Robinia pseudacacia**

BLOATING AND FLATULENCE

The reason for a bloated feeling or experiencing flatulence is often food that is difficult to digest or is unfamiliar; for example, certain kinds of vegetables cause gas to build up (cabbage, onions, leeks) or are less digestible (like fresh bread, yeast products, and dried fruit). But such problems can also be due to emotional stress. IMPORTANT: If the symptoms do not improve in spite of self-treatment or a change in diet, seek advice from an experienced homeopath.

KEY SYMPTOMS	REMEDY
Heavy feeling; burping tastes like undigested food; weak stomach; thick white coating on the tongue; can't handle baked goods, pork, tea, nicotine, or sour food.	**Antimonium crudum**
Feeling stuffed; sour burping of undigested food; abdomen visibly bloated; passing foul-smelling gas but has no relief; gas starts while still eating; craves sour foods, sweets, strong alcoholic beverages, coffee, and cold water. *Worse:* milk, tea, fruit	**China**
Bloated stomach; passing gas and rancid-tasting burping brings relief; bloated and lethargic; particularly after heavy meals of meat, cabbage, legumes, milk, coffee, and wine. *Worse:* after eating, tight clothes, lying down *Better:* fresh air	**Carbo vegetabilis**
Visibly bloated abdomen below the navel, specifically on the left side; distinct sounds in the intestine on the left side; good appetite but full after only a few bites (then feels stuffed) or wants to eat constantly. Especially for those who are mentally active, choleric, and aged before their years.	**Lycopodium D12**

KEY SYMPTOMS	REMEDY
Feels stuffed immediately after eating; slowly increasing flatulence, must loosen belt and unbutton pants/skirt; extremely tired 2 hours after a meal; craving for stimulants like coffee, tea, and alcohol. Especially for ambitious, choleric, and pedantic people.	**Nux vomica** **D12**
Flatulence with colic-like pain; loud stomach and intestinal noises; food sits in the stomach like a rock; burping tastes rancid; can't tolerate fatty foods; can't tolerate pork, fruit, ice cream, baked goods; occurs when eating too many different food at once. Especially for people who are moody and emotionally needy.	**Pulsatilla** **D12**
Constant feeling of being stuffed; constant flatulence; passing foul-smelling gas (smells like rotten eggs); the whole abdomen visibly bloated; colic-like pain; loud stomach and intestinal noises; sometimes diarrhea in the morning. *Worse:* in the evening, during the night	**Sulfur**

SLUGGISHNESS AND CONSTIPATION

The usual cause of this kind of complaint is a sedentary lifestyle, eating fatty foods, and the misuse of laxatives. Preventive measures include fiber-rich food with ample amounts of raw vegetables and liquids, movement, and exercise. IMPORTANT: If the individual has been on a laxative over a prolonged period of time (including herbal teas and fruit-based remedies), seek advice from an experienced homeopath.

KEY SYMPTOMS	REMEDY
Unsuccessful attempts to produce stool even after heavy pushing; ravenous appetite; cannot tolerate potatoes. Especially for those who sit too much. *Worse:* cold, during the winter	**Alumina**
Constipation; stool is hard, then paste-like. Especially for lethargic children and young people with weight problems and aversions to sports, meat, and cooked food. *Worse:* cold/damp, work *Better:* warmth, lying down	**Calcarea carbonica**
Feels stuffed; has a visibly bloated stomach, but is unable to burp; passes foul-smelling gas; stool is hard and knotted and causes painful, bleeding tears in the rectum. Especially for people with weight problems.	**Graphites**
Cramps, extreme flatulence; feels constipated in spite of having passed stool; good appetite, but full after only a few bites or can't get enough. Especially for mentally active, choleric people and those who look to have aged prematurely.	**Lycopodium D12**
Sluggish intestine and constipation due to misuse of laxatives; feels extremely stuffed after eating; thick coating on the tongue; bad breath; has an aversion to eating in the morning.	**Nux vomica D12**

CHAPTER 7

THE KIDNEYS AND THE URINARY TRACT

PAINFUL KIDNEYS AND KIDNEY COLIC

The reason for serious, persistent pain in the kidneys is usually a kidney or pelvic infection that originally started out in the urethra and bladder. Symptoms of this type of infection include shivers, fever, and blood in the urine. However, if there is a wave-like pain that lessens after about 5 to 7 hours, the cause of the pain is most likely kidney stones. Generally speaking, seek medical help immediately for any kidney pain. The following remedies are meant to relieve the pain and thereby make waiting for the appointment a little easier. NOTE: If kidney problems occur frequently, see an experienced homeopath for constitutional therapy.

KEY SYMPTOMS	REMEDY
Kidney stones are affected by changes in the weather; colic-like pain when weather changes and also during fog. Especially for people who tend toward rheumatism and gout and are very sensitive to cold. *Worse:* cold, motion, warm bed *Better:* warm rooms	**Acidum formicicum**
Sudden, severe throbbing pain, radiating into lower abdomen (urethra) and sides; highly sensitive to motion; face hot, sweaty, flushed; feet, later hands often cold; an acute anxiety attack. *Worse:* cold, motion *Better:* warmth (warm bed), rest/quiet	**Belladonna D6***
Burning, stabbing, localized pain, particularly on left side; radiates far into thighs and knees; sometimes almost causes fainting because of severity of pain; highly sensitive to motion; urine is sparse, has red sediment. *Worse:* motion, pressure *Better:* warmth, rest/quiet	**Berberis**

*One dose every 30 minutes until better; or 1 dose every 15 minutes, but not more than 5 doses.

KEY SYMPTOMS	REMEDY
Severe burning, stabbing, or tearing pain in the kidneys or bladder that, for men, may radiate into the penis; unbearable, constant pressure in the bladder; urine produced in drops only. *Worse:* cold water, coffee	**Cantharis**
Severe, cramp-like, tearing pain; patient doubles over; frequent urge to urinate accompanied by burning pain; urine sparse with red sediment; also has urge to urinate but cannot produce urine; occurs especially when worry "hits" the kidneys. *Better:* doubled over, bending down, warmth	**Colocynthis**
Cramp-like, stabbing pain radiates into the bladder; unbearable pressure on the bladder; often has urges to urinate but cannot produce urine; urine sparse, has red sediment; particularly when passes brick-colored "sand" from the left kidney. *Worse:* when waking up, touch, pressure *Better:* walking, warmth	**Coccus cacti**
Cramp-like, shooting, localized pain, particularly on the right side; radiates into the abdomen/pelvic area, legs, less often arms; extensive stretching relieves pain; has cold sweats. *Worse:* in the evening, nights, lying down, doubling over, pressure *Better:* stretching, walking	**Dioscorea**
Painful urge to urinate but cannot produce urine; burning and tearing sensation in the bladder and urethra. *Worse:* cold, after rage, anger *Better:* warmth	**Nux vomica D12**

CYSTITIS

This bladder catarrh or infection is usually due to a bacterial inflammation of the urethra, often affecting the bladder and kidneys. Most often it is a case of having become chilled, being pregnant, and/or having poor hygiene. But a nonbacterial irritation of the urethra is also possible, and this can be due to clothing that is too tight; it can be caused by unfamiliar, intense sexual intercourse; or the irritation can occur as a "by-product" of passing kidney "sand." To prevent cystitis, drink plenty of fluids and wear "breathable" underwear (avoid pads with a plastic liner). IMPORTANT: See your physician immediately if there is a persistent problem, high fever (102° F/39° C), or in the presence of bloody or purulent urine.

Self-treatment is acceptable during pregnancy only after consulting with your homeopath or midwife.

KEY SYMPTOMS	REMEDY
"Stormy" beginning; unbearable burning pain with constant urges to urinate; urine is hot, sparse, sometimes reddish in color; person has shivers; is extremely thirsty for cold water; deathly afraid, very restless; particularly when urinating; often due to cold, dry wind, or draft when driving a car. *Worse:* warmth in any form, nights, warm rooms *Better:* after sweating	**Aconitum D12*/****
Stabbing, burning pain when urinating, particularly at the very end; urge to urinate with a constant feeling of pressure; produces little urine, often dark in color; not very thirsty; warmth and tight clothing all of a sudden can't be tolerated. *Worse:* warmth in any form, pressure *Better:* fresh air	**Apis mellifica**

*Every 30 minutes until improvement sets in, but not more than 5 doses.
**If experienced, 1 or 3 doses of C30.

KEY SYMPTOMS	REMEDY
Sudden onset; the whole body feels feverish and hot while feet are often cold; head feels hot, pupils are dilated; burning pain in the bladder; urge to urinate without producing urine; usually due to having become chilled. *Worse:* cold, motion, vibration *Better:* warmth (warm bed), rest/quiet	**Belladonna D6***
Constant urge to urinate, with unbearable burning and stabbing pain; biting pain in the bladder; urine is produced only in little drops; very hot and cloudy; severe thirst but has either an aversion to drinking or an unquenchable thirst. *Worse:* cold water, coffee	**Cantharis**
Painful urge to urinate, particularly when cold; burning pain at the opening of the urethra when urinating; urine cloudy and slimy; usually due to having become chilled or wet in summer or late fall. *Better:* warmth in any form	**Dulcamara**
Extreme urge to urinate; stabbing, burning pain when urinating, particularly at the opening and around the urethra; pain of longer duration; unusual night perspiration that is foul-smelling. *Worse:* nights, change in temperature	**Mercurius solubilis D12**
Main remedy for irritated bladder due to having become chilled or drinking too much beer or fruit juice; frequent, painful urges to urinate but little urine is produced; very nervous and irritated; sensitive to cold. *Worse:* cold, draft, coffee, mental stress *Better:* warmth in any form, rest/quiet	**Nux vomica**

*Every 30 minutes until improvement sets in, but no more than 5 doses.

KEY SYMPTOMS	REMEDY
Painful bladder irritation, sometimes with a cramp-like sensation just before urination that radiates into the thighs; urge to urinate after having urinated; not very thirsty; often caused by the feet having become chilled and wet. Especially for people who are moody and tend to whine. *Better:* fresh air, receiving sympathy	**Pulsatilla D12**
Frequent urge to urinate, with severe burning sensation or totally pain-free; plenty of light-colored urine; urinating is easier while standing.	**Sarsaparilla**
Frequent urges to urinate, but urine does not flow immediately and is foul-smelling. *Worse:* after intercourse, cold *Better:* warmth	**Sepia**

CHAPTER 8

WOMEN'S HEALTH

BASIC INFORMATION

Being attractive and productive is, to a large extent in our culture, considered to be synonymous with being young. This attitude has caused women and men, in ever increasing numbers, to worry and fear that they are past their prime and are failing to satisfy the requirements and the demands made on them. Such pressure, in the long run, will influence the well-being and health of a person to a great degree.

Women often carry double and triple burdens: raising children and caring for the needs of the family or household as well as maintaining their job responsibilities. Many, particularly single women, simply must work full-time for financial reasons. Others may remain in their chosen profession or work so as not to lose seniority, health care, or job qualifications, and some simply continue working because rejoining the work force later is often very difficult. Women of every age, but especially between the ages of 25 and 45, accomplish a tremendous amount of work, day in and day out.

But even that does not tell whole story: they are also dealing with the tremendous pressure of having to be perfect—always the perfect housewife and mother, perfect partner, perfect colleague. It is well known that all this seems to works out rather well for a while. But sooner or later, a person's reserves get used up, and it makes life even more difficult when one starts to feel not quite okay, nervous, depressed, and in pain.

For women, many of these complaints are closely tied to their menstrual cycle and reproductive organs. As annoying and bothersome as the above-mentioned symptoms may be, they can be seen as a helpful message, making a woman aware that her energy reserves are low and that it is essential to take a break to "recharge the battery." What form such a break should take is different from one women to another: one might need more sleep (the main problem for mothers, by the way), others may need to take a long vacation or visit a spa. However, this is, generally speaking, not enough. Most women must learn to take themselves more seriously. This means, for instance, reducing the desire for perfection and the amount of work, delegating some of the family and household chores to a partner and children, organizing a support system among neighbors, and so on. The list of possibilities is long, and every woman must figure out what will work best to handle her own personal situation.

Here, too, homeopathy can provide valuable support. The proper remedy can activate a woman's self-healing capacity and make sure that her physical and mental/emotional balance is restored, allowing her to go about her daily life free from pain and fatigue, all of which makes it easier to separate what is essential from that which is less important.

Of course, here, too, self-treatment is subject to all the general rules we have discussed before: only nonsevere, acute complaints should be "self-treated." Those complaints of longer duration or those that seem to occur frequently need the care and/or advice of an experienced physician or homeopath.

See your gynecologist if:

- you have a problem during your pregnancy
- in case of heavy or unusual bleeding (heavy clots, pieces of tissue)
- bleeding between regular periods
- bleeding after menopause
- vaginal discharge
- sudden, severe pain in the lower abdomen
- all types of abdomenal problems involving fever
- visible or noticeable swelling in the area of the abdomen
- unspecified pain in the abdomen, also pain during intercourse
- abdominal injuries
- changes in the area of the breast, nipples, underarm (swelling, lumps, tissue that seems to be pulled in, sudden discharge from the nipples)
- if the last gynecological examination was more then 6 month ago

When in doubt, always see your physician.

IMPORTANT: Self-treatment with homeopathic remedies can never replace breast self-examination as well as regular gynecological examination.

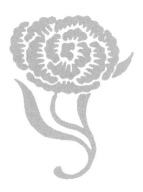

PREMENSTRUAL PROBLEMS

The main problems prior to the onset of menstruation—also called premenstrual syndrome (PMS)—are nervousness, sadness, headaches, pain in the abdomen, water retention, and sensitive breasts. These symptoms are caused by the cyclical fluctuation of hormone production. See also Chapters 1 and 2. Dosage: a standard dose, D12, once a day until improvement sets in, but over no more than two cycles.

KEY SYMPTOMS	REMEDY
Tired, depressed, shy; water retention, particularly in the feet, feeling as heavy as lead; joint pain; hands and feet are ice-cold. *Worse:* in the morning, cold *Better:* eating, motion, onset of menstruation	**Aristolochia**
Headaches; painful, swollen breasts; cramps; depressed; self-doubt; cold/damp sweats; quickly exhausted. Particularly for motherly types with a tendency to being overweight. *Worse:* cold, dampness/humidity	**Calcarea carbonica**
Depressed; irritated; cries easily; breasts are sensitive; feet swollen; lower body and back pain; diarrhea at the onset of menstruation; an aversion to sex. *Worse:* since being pregnant	**Causticum**
Head and neck pain, often on the left side; sad; nervous; rushing; always in motion; keeps talking about self all the time or does not care; better at the onset of menstruation; pain tearing from one side of the hip to the other; the heavier the bleeding, the more severe the pain. *Better:* warmth	**Cimicifuga**
Constantly under pressure, irritated, and restless; headaches, migraines, including	**Lachesis**

dizziness and nosebleeds; cramps and back pain;
the heavier the bleeding, the more severe the pain;
can't stand anything tight around neck and body.
Worse: warmth of any kind

Frightened, sad; shy; is always close to tears; also   **Lycopodium**
tyrannical and unkind; self-doubt; cramps;
visibly bloated, passing gas does not bring relief;
ravenous for sweets and spicy food.
Worse: warmth, tight clothes

Head aches as if it is going to burst; introverted   **Natrum**
behavior; moody; a tendency to dramatize; easily   **chloratum**
exhausted; absent-minded.
Worse: before noon, heat, receiving sympathy
Better: salt, fresh air, being alone

Nausea, heartburn; breast and stomach painful;   **Nux vomica**
very nervous; choleric; dissatisfied; egocentric;
believes that accomplishment is what counts;
feels annoyed and restricted by menstruation;
strong libido.
Worse: in the morning, cold
Better: warmth

Very sensitive, cries easily; moody; good-   **Pulsatilla**
natured; free-spirited; headaches; pulling
sensation in the uterus; onset of menstruation
often delayed and scant.
Worse: warmth
Better: fresh air; receiving sympathy

Headaches, cramps; discharge causing a rash;   **Sepia**
totally exhausted; overworked; feeling of
emptiness; suddenly appearing rage and tears;
very conscientious.
Worse: during menstruation, cold
Better: warmth, light motion, rest/quiet

PAINFUL MENSTRUATION

Painful menstruation is caused by hormone fluctuation, a tumor, the abnormal growth of the tissues in the uterus (endomitriosis), or surgical scars (after a cesarean section, for instance). But emotional stress can also be responsible. Before starting self-treatment, check with your physician. In addition to the remedies listed under Premenstrual Problems, the following remedies have also been proven to be effective. Dosage: If in severe pain, take one standard dose every 15 minutes in the potency indicated until symptoms improve, but no more than 6 times.

KEY SYMPTOMS	REMEDY
Stabbing pain and cramps just immediately prior to and during menstruation; often pounding, hot headaches/migraine, particularly on the right side; bleeding too heavy, too early or too late, light red with lumps, warm, and bad-smelling; the person is very thirsty. *Worse:* motion, vibration	**Belladonna D6**
Bladder and intestinal cramps, pain moving back and forth; headaches, particularly in the first two days; the less the bleeding, the more severe the pain.	**Caulophyllum D6**
Unbearable colic shortly before and during menstruation that radiates extensively throughout; hot sweating spells; nausea; vomiting; heavy bleeding with clots; very restless; bad tempered. *Worse:* when angry *Better:* walking around	**Chamomilla D12**
Cramps before and during menstruation; surface of the stomach very sensitive to touch; definite weakness; bleeding too heavy, too dark, lumpy. *Worse:* lack of sleep	**Cocculus D6**

KEY SYMPTOMS	REMEDY
Sharp wave-like attacks of pain that cause doubling over; internally very nervous, restless; often after anger. Especially for those with ovarian cysts. *Better:* bending over, warmth	**Colocynthis D6**
Very stressed, even minor pain becomes unbearable; bleeds too early, for too long, and shows a light or dark red color, lumpy; severe vaginal itching, increased libido; very sensitive to noises and smells. *Worse:* excitement, coffee, motion	**Coffea D12**
Pain at the onset of bleeding; bleeding too early and too heavy, lumpy. Especially for women who are full of sadness and contradictions.	**Ignatia D12**
Cramps and colic, even during the night; bleeds too early, dark, and stringy; very weak, barely able to walk. *Better:* warmth, pressure, onset of bleeding	**Magnesium phosphoricum D6**
Severe cramps or dull pain radiating into the thighs and back; bleeding late and sparsely, and producing a foul odor; often only for a few hours; also when there may have been a previous (possibly undetected) miscarriage. *Worse:* early in the morning	**Viburnum D6**
Extremely severe cramps affecting the circulatory system; the person shivers, has cold sweat on forehead; dizziness, nausea; vomits until collapses; often diarrhea; extremely weak.	**Veratrum album D6**

HEAVY MENSTRUATION

See the previous section, Painful Menstruation. Many of the recommended remedies under that heading are also helpful for heavy menstruation and vice versa. Before starting a self-treatment program, check with your physician. ATTENTION: Heavy bleeding may cause anemia; have the level of the iron* in your blood tested.

Dosage: 1 standard dose daily in the potency indicated until improvement sets in, but at a maximum of two cycles only. In acute situations, take a standard dose every 15 minutes until symptoms improve, but no more than 6 times.

KEY SYMPTOMS	REMEDY
Bleeding starts too early, too heavy; with pain "pushing downward"; depressed; has a pale complexion with a tendency to have anemia.	**Agnus castus D6**
Bleeds too early, too long; menses is lumpy and cream-like; the slightest excitement worsens the symptoms; sharp pain in the lower abdomen; very weak, dizzy; catches a cold easily; has toothaches. *Worse:* cold, dampness	**Calcarea carbonica D12**
Bleeds too early, too late, and spasmodically; menses is dark and lumpy; abdomen is bloated with cramps; has headaches with dizziness; a pale complexion; is very weak and nervous. *Better:* warmth	**China D4**
Bleeds light red, spasmodically, particularly when moving; cramps in the bladder.	**Erigon D1–D3**

*Homeopathic remedies can be helpful in rectifying iron deficiences but should be given in combination with specific iron preparations.

KEY SYMPTOMS	REMEDY
Menses is dark, coagulated; pain in the surface of the abdomen, back, and pelvis; cramps during menstruation, but also pain and bleeding between the cycles.	**Hamamelis D2–D4**
Bleeds too early, too long; menses is thin watery, and foul-smelling, causing rashes and itching; sharp abdominal pain, backache, and periodic sweating. *Worse:* exhaustion, after having given birth *Better:* sitting down, pressure	**Kali carbonicum D6**
Bleeds too early, too long; menses is light red and watery; congestion in the head and dizziness, particularly after heavy lifting.	**Millefolium D4**
Bleeds too early, too long; less often too late; also accompanied by anemia. Especially for pale, nervous women with light hair, who have a tendency to bruise easily.	**Phosphorus D6 or D12**
Bleeds too early and spasmodically when moving; menses is either too light or too dark in color; useful in cases of endomitriosis. Especially for women who gain weight easily. *Worse:* excitement, anger	**Sabina D2-D3**

PROBLEMS DURING PREGNANCY

When pregnant, always check with your physician or homeopath when-ever physical, mental, or emotional complaints appear. Only morning sickness and constipation may be self-treated. For varicose veins or hem-orrhoids, see Chapter 9. But here, too, the advice is that you self-treat only after consulting with your physician or midwife.

KEY SYMPTOMS	REMEDY
Ravenously hungry, afterward nausea to the point of fainting; burning, ice-cold sensation and pain in the stomach; flatulence; restless; nervous; hasty; exhausted. *Worse:* seeing/smelling food, particularly fish	Colchicum D4
Overly sensitive to tobacco smoke; sometimes has an aversion to something, sometimes not. *Worse:* when stomach is empty	Ignatia D12
Constantly nauseated, vomiting does not bring relief; strong urges for sweets; tongue is clear; moody, indecisive. *Worse:* in the evening, night, after a heavy meal; motion, bending down *Better:* cold drinks, fresh air, rest/quiet	Ipecacuanha D6
Nausea, vomiting, or vomiting after eating, particularly in the morning; stomach pressure; food sits in the stomach like a rock; nosebleeds. Especially for women who are action-oriented and react to any interruption in their plans with annoyance and anger, or those who are unable to do without coffee, nicotine, and alcohol. *Worse:* in the morning, smells, noise, bright light	Nux vomica D12

KEY SYMPTOMS	REMEDY

Strong aversion to fat while having attacks
of ravenous urges for fatty food, and suffering
afterward from nausea, heartburn, heavyj
stomach; bitter taste in the mouth, not very
thirsty; very emotional, changeable moods.
Worse: eating in the evening, heavy food, warmth
Better: fresh air, receiving sympathy

Pulsatilla D12

Morning sickness is worse when smelling
food; at times insatiably hungry; ravenous
urges for something sour; aversion to meat
and milk; often constipated; sudden outbursts
of anger and tears.
Better: light movements, rest/quiet, being
alone, lying down on the right side

Sepia D12

Heartburn and stomach pain after eating;
strong aversion to warm meals; is asking for
cold food and cold water; indecisive; worries
a lot for no apparent reason.
Worse: excitement

Silicea D12

Nausea and vomiting affects the circulatory
system: dizziness, cold sweat on the forehead,
pale complexion, body ice-cold; feels very
sick; needs to loosen clothing.
Worse: in the morning, traveling in car/train/ship
Better: fresh air

Tabacum D6

PREPARING FOR A BIRTH

Homeopathy offers numerous remedies that can make a birth easier. Most of them serve to keep the musculature elastic, to relieve muscle spasm in the pelvic area as well as lessen the (absolutely normal) fear prior to giving birth. Dealing with all the above makes a birth much less stressful and less painful. The choice of the proper remedies is not only guided by the prevailing pain but also, and very specifically, by the overall physical and mental/emotional situation of the mother-to-be. It is therefore recommended to let an experienced homeopath and the attending midwife choose the remedy.

NOTE: Since remedies are usually taken several weeks before the birth takes place, make sure you consult your homeopath early.

If it is impossible to get professional advice or if time is short, self-treatment is better than none at all. Here, two remedies from the homeopathic medicine chest are particularly effective. One is *Pulsatilla* D12: to balance the emotional state and to give strength to the mother; and the second is *Arnica* C30: to prepare for the enormous physical stress during the actual birthing process and to avoid bleeding.

IMPORTANT: Inform your attending physician and midwife in the clinic about what you have been using.

- *Pulsatilla* D12: Begin taking this remedy about 4 to 6 weeks prior to the expected date; 1 standard dose daily.
- *Arnica* C30: One standard dose when the contractions begin—possibly repeated one more time—as well as 1 to 2 doses after the birth.

If you feel particularly physically tense, consider taking *Caulophyllum* D6 2 to 3 weeks prior to the expected date three times daily, alternating every day with *Pulsatilla*.

PROBLEMS AFTER THE BIRTH

The recommendations given for "before a birth" also hold for the treatment of problems that appear afterward. Self-treatment should only be attempted if professional advice is not available. But an experienced homeopath should be consulted as soon as possible. IMPORTANT: In case of severe pain, fever, or bleeding, seek medical help immediately.

The following remedies have been helpful in lessening pain and in supporting the healing process after the birth:

◻ *Arnica* C30: Two standard doses, the first 3 hours after the birth, the second 12 hours later. Also after forced birth, vacuum procedure, or a torn perineum.
◻ *Bellis perennis* D12: For severe pain in the uterus, similar to a bruising, mix one standard dose in a glass of water and drink in small sips until symptoms improve.
◻ *Hypericum* D12: Especially after tearing of the perineum, one standard dose to be taken 3 times daily.
◻ *Staphysagria* D12: For severe pain, particularly after a cesarean, mix one standard dose in a half glass of water and take in small sips until symptoms improve.

To lessen the after-effects of anesthesia, including local injection (epidural) or other pain-controlling medication:

◻ *Nux vomica* D12: Mix one standard dose in a half glass of water and drink in small sips until symptoms improve.

For postpartum depression, baby-blues, "crying jags":

◻ *Pulsatilla* D12: Once daily, a standard dose.

If there are more severe complaints, increased restlessness, and strange emotional sensations, seek advice immediately from your physician or call your midwife. Explain the problem as precisely as you can, because you might be dealing with postnatal confusion, which can be easily treated, if attended to promptly. Here, too, homeopathic remedies have proven to be very helpful.

NURSING PROBLEMS

The most common problems while nursing are a slow-down in the production of milk, painful irritations or injuries to the nipple, and infection of the breasts. If the difficulty has not improved after one day of self-treatment, seek homeopathic advice (a physician or midwife). ATTENTION: Treating breast infections should be attempted only in the very beginning stages and, even then, only by an experienced lay person. With fever, severe pain, and inflammation of the breast, take one of the following remedies and see your physician immediately.

KEY SYMPTOMS	REMEDY
Breast infection; sudden, stabbing pain in the breasts, skin is hot, sweaty and red; often accompanied by headaches. *Worse:* motion, vibration	**Belladonna D6***
Breast infection; breasts are very hard and heavy, with stabbing pain; very sensitive to touch, slightly inflamed; often accompanied by extreme thirst. *Worse:* slightest movement *Better:* consistent, firm pressure	**Bryonia D12**
Nipple very sensitive, sore, and cracked; flow of milk fluctuating—at times too little, at other times too much; skin is damp/cold but breasts are hot, swollen; easily exhausted. Especially for women with weight problems. *Worse:* cold	**Calcarea carbonica D12**
Nipples are highly sensitive, clothing cannot be tolerated; severe pain into the back when the baby is nursing; breasts also hard and swollen.	**Croton tiglium D6**

*Every ½ to 2 hours until improvement begins.

KEY SYMPTOMS	REMEDY
Milk-flow reduced after anger and agitation.	**Ignatia D12**
Very sensitive to vibration; pain is constant; can hardly walk, must hold breasts; also for breast infection. *Worse:* cold, motion	**Lac caninum D12**
Nipples are sore, cracked, often bloody, painful, particularly when nursing; breaks into heavy sweat at the slightest exertion. *Worse:* nights *Better:* rest/quiet	**Mercurius solubilis D12**
Nipples are sensitive, sore, with aching pain when nursing. Especially for action-oriented women who react to interference with impatience and annoyance.	**Nux vomica D12**
Breasts are very hard, hot, swollen, very painful; pain throughout whole body while nursing; nipples are very sensitive, sore, often with small cracks/ulcers; also for breast infections.	**Phytolacca D12**
Nipples and breasts are sore, sensitive; painful breasts, radiating alternatively into the back, abdomen, and head; she starts to cry suddenly while nursing; also a good remedy for reduction in milk flow due to mood swings. *Worse:* warmth	**Pulsatilla D12**
Nipples are very sensitive, sore with deep cracks; when beginning to nurse, intense contractions of the uterus and slight bleeding.	**Silicea D6**
Nipples are cracked, frayed, and sore, with burning pain, particularly after nursing, radiating into the back; also for reduction in milk production. *Worse:* nights; washing	**Sulfur D6**

MENOPAUSAL PROBLEMS

The most common problems during menopause are hot flashes accompanied by perspiration, nervousness, depression, anxiety, dry skin (including soft tissue), irregular, heavy, and painful menstruation, and bone loss (osteoporosis). The reasons for these syptoms are manifold: hormonal changes and the result of everyday stress over many decades. But other momentous changes, like children leaving the "nest," can also play a role. Many women in this phase of their lives have time to themselves for the first time in years but are reluctant to make use of it. Since menopause, similar to puberty, represents a fundamental life change, it is recommended to consult an experienced homeopath as a matter of course. Many are also encouraged to undergo a constitutional therapy at this time. In the interim, and only if the above-mentioned difficulties are minor (they usually show up together), the following remedies can be helpful. Also check under the terms/chapters elsewhere in this book where these difficulties are also discussed.

Dosage: If not indicated otherwise: in case of predominately physical complaints D6, 3 times daily; if the complaints are more emotional and of a nervous type, D12, once daily until symptoms improve; however, at most, take the remedy only for two cycles or 8 weeks.

KEY SYMPTOMS	REMEDY
Periodically under nervous pressure; restless; confused; anxious; fear of becoming sick; depressed; without joy; in a hurry, always on the move; talks all the time or is listless; hot flashes without perspiration; shooting headaches and nerve pain, migraine; tension in the neck, particularly on the left side; empty sensation in the stomach but no appetite; irregular bleeding with wave-like pain. *Worse:* mornings, damp/cold weather, menstruating *Better:* warmth, being outside, small meals	**Cimicifuga**
Has constant nervous tension, irritated, restless; needs to talk all the time; suspicious, jealous; depressed, anxious; hot flashes, perspiration	**Lachesis D12**

with strong odor, constantly sweaty; feels
physically weak; heart palpitations; headaches,
migraines with dizziness and nosebleeds,
particularly on the left side; irregular and heavy
menstruation with cramps, backache; can't
stand tight things around the neck and body.
Worse: warmth of any type, humid/warm
weather, wine, after sleeping
Better: onset of menstruation

Introverted, sad, serious, unforgiving, moody;   **Natrum**
tends to dramatize; constantly thinks about   **chloratum**
old hurts but resents kindness; wants to be
left alone, but cries when alone; can't sleep
because of worry; depressed, anxious, fearful,
is afraid of making a fool of herself; heart
palpitations and fear when in a small place
and among people; has tendency to faint; is
easily exhausted; a pale complexion; tends to be
anemic; sacrifices for others; excruciating
headaches/migraine; itching around the genitalia;
vaginal dryness; painful sex; irregular, heavy
menstruation.
Worse: in the P.M., heat, noise, receiving sympathy
Better: fresh air, being outdoors, when left alone

Very sensitive with constantly changing moods;   **Pulsatilla D12**
worries about others but needs much attention
herself; complaining, suspicious, jealous, sad,
whiny and then again turning gentle, happy,
good-natured, and carefree; afraid particularly of
the dark, the future, and being alone; nervous
headache; pale with a tendency to anemia; constant
sweating all over the body; uterus prolapse;
rheumatic complaints.
Worse: warmth in any form
Better: fresh air, outdoors, motion, attention,
receiving sympathy

KEY SYMPTOMS	REMEDY

Totally exhausted, overworked; inner   **Sepia**
emptiness and feeling burned out, abandoned,
helpless, anxious; does not care about family
and job; sudden outbursts of anger and tears;
hot flashes and outbreaks of cold sweat;
yellowish-pale complexion with dark circles;
often headaches/migraines; continues working
only due to a sense of responsibility; menstruation
is irregular, too long, smells bad, and causes rashes;
often accompanied by headaches and cramps;
feeling of downward pressure; uterus prolapse;
aversion to sex.
Worse: mornings, evenings, when menstruating,
cold
Better: warmth, moderate movemen, being
outdoors, when alone, rest/quiet

Self-absorbed, has mood swings; active,   **Sulfur**
impatient; makes many plans, then becomes
depressed again with no drive; frequently
needs to bend over; hot flashes with perspiration,
leading to severe exhaustion; attacks of perspiring
fromthe head, hands, and feet; palm of hands
and soles of feet are hot and burning when in bed;
sticks feet out from under the covers; itching and
soreness of the external genitalia; nausea, dizziness,
and diarrhea in the morning; tendency to have
back and bladder pain in the morning; has heavy
legs and varicose veins.
Worse: in the morning, water, standing, heat,
exertion
Better: many small meals, sweets, lying down

CHAPTER 9

VENOUS PROBLEMS

VARICOSE VEINS

Varicose veins develop when a vein's wall becomes stretched, and the venous valves fail to close properly, preventing the blood from flowing freely throughout the system. When this happens, some of the blood is left behind, and the vein becomes clogged. This problem is often hereditary but can also develop from increased pressure on the blood vessels in the abdomen during pregnancy or because of being overweight. Measures to counteract varicose veins are regular exercise, moving from heels to toes while standing, and elevating the legs when sitting. The diagnosis should be made by your physician.

Timely treatment with homeopathic remedies can prevent varicose veins, but the discomfort of those already existing can most certainly be reduced. When varicose veins run in the family and are accompanied by constipation (with hemorrhoids), or when the remedies listed do not bring relief after 6 weeks, a constitutional therapy supervised by an experienced homeopath is advised. IMPORTANT: Self-treat during pregnancy *only* after consultation with your physician or midwife! If varicose veins are inflamed and cause severe pain or swelling, see your physician immediately. There is always danger of a developing thrombosis!

KEY SYMPTOMS	REMEDY
Red and blue varicose veins; ulcers surrounded by dark red circles; particularly during pregnancy with hemorrhoids appearing simultaneously; everything is moving at slow speed. IMPORTANT: *Aesculus* is not effective in the presence of inflammation. *Worse:* walking *Better:* warm weather	**Aesculus**
Heavy, stiff legs, often feeling as if paralyzed; legs "fall asleep" easily; a feeling of cold from the knee downward; tired and weak with a tendency to faint, often with digestive problems and flatulence. *Better:* fresh air, fanning	**Carbo vegetabilis**

KEY SYMPTOMS	REMEDY
Varicose veins, particularly in the lower leg; legs are heavy, tired, swollen, and feel as if they were bruised; sharp, stabbing, or prickly pain. Especially for women with pregnancy-related varicose veins and hemorrhoids at the same time. *Worse:* warmth, humidity	**Hamamelis**
Tired, heavy legs, often with swelling in the knee area; must elevate legs, otherwise severe pain; legs "fall asleep" easily when standing, often with stabbing pains during the night. *Worse:* warmth in any form *Better:* moderate movement outdoors	**Pulsatilla**
Very large varicose veins; legs and feet are restless, must move them constantly; muscles are jittery and twitch; cramps in the lower legs; feelings of numbness and numb spots, particularly in the lower legs; especially for varicose veins that have become worse during pregnancy and during menopause.	**Zincum metallicum**

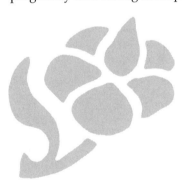

HEMORRHOIDS

Hemorrhoids are really varicose veins in the rectum. The symptoms are pain, burning, itching, and bright-red bleeding when eliminating. General recommendations are as follows: assure regularity, not with laxatives, but rather with a fiber-rich diet that includes a sufficient amount of raw vegetables and whole-wheat products, with the possible addition of wheat germ. Do not eat very spicy or sour foods, and do not consume coffee. Drink plenty of fluids. Observe careful hygiene to avoid infections. After each elimination, clean the rectum with clear water.

The diagnosis should always be made by a physician, who must decide—when there are severe complaints—if the hemorrhoids should be removed surgically. If the remedies listed below (also available in the form of creams for external application) do not improve symptoms within 6 weeks, or if laxatives were taken over a longer period of time, a constitutional therapy should be considered. IMPORTANT: Avoid self-treatment during pregnancy until after you have consulted with your physician or midwife.

KEY SYMPTOMS	REMEDY
Burning, stabbing pain, radiating into the back, and not only at the time of elimination; often accompanied by constipation (change your diet); almost no bleeding; burning sensation in the rectum; itching; dryness, heat. *Worse:* during elimination, walking *Better:* warm weather	**Aesculus**
Severe pain; rectum feels sore or bruised, often inflamed; constant bleeding during elimination; intense, hot itching with cramps in the rectum; often accompanied by chronic constipation (change your diet!); also in cases of pregnancy-related hemorrhoids.	**Hamamelis**

CHAPTER 10

CHILDHOOD ILLNESSES

BASIC INFORMATION

Classical childhood illnesses like measles, mumps, German measles, chicken pox, and whooping cough can be "self-treated," generally speaking. The diagnosis, however, must be made by your physician. Because of the danger of infection, it is important to phone ahead for the appointment. While scarlet fever also belongs to the same category of childhood diseases, it must be treated by a physician because of a high potential for complications.

In homeopathy, each childhood illness is assigned a specific remedy that, if given in the early stages, can lessen the severity as well as the duration of the disease. For instance, *Pertussinum* is for whooping cough, *Morbillinum* for measles, and *Variolinum* for chicken pox. These remedies are produced from germs and can only be used by a physician. If, therefore, an infectious disease is making "its rounds," and a child shows some of the first signs of that particular infection—like a visibly pale complexion, listlessness, increased irritability, etc.—see your homeopath or physician immediately.

Babies and small children under the age of 2 should always and only be treated by your physician; do not attempt treatment yourself. Too, keep in mind that childhood diseases, when they affect adults, can become very serious. In such cases, always consult your physician!

See your physician immediately if you notice any of the following:

¤ feeling extremely bad, tired, and weak
¤ high fever (102° F/39° C)
¤ head and ear pain or difficulty hearing, particularly in the case of mumps
¤ abdominal aches, particularly in the case of mumps
¤ severe coughing and/or heavy mucus buildup of the bronchial tubes, particularly in cases of measles and whooping cough

If any of the following occur, seek immediate medical treatment in your physician's office or at an emergency room:

¤ severe headaches with nausea and vomiting
¤ stiff neck
¤ difficulty in breathing, suspecting pneumonia (the sides of the nose vibrate with every breath)
¤ persistent cramps, lips turning bluish
¤ persistent cramps with fever
¤ feeling dazed, showing confusion, fainting

CHICKEN POX

Chicken pox is a highly infectious disease that occurs primarily in school-age children. Incubation time is roughly 2 to 3 weeks. Usually there is only a slight elevation in temperature. Lentil-size red patches appear on the skin and, within a few hours, become very itchy and produce watery blisters. Sometimes only a few spots are present, but frequently the rash covers the whole body. All in all, chicken pox is not a severe illness, and homeopathic remedies can reduce the itching, prevent infection, and speed up the healing of blisters. IMPORTANT: If the blisters become infected or if other complications should arise (see previous page), see your physician immediately!

KEY SYMPTOMS	REMEDY
Turbulent or sudden onset with rapidly rising temperature, but no skin rash yet. For symptoms/dosages see Viral Infection (Flu), page 70.	**Aconitum D12** or **Belladonna D6**
Small blisters in the oral cavity and the area of the genitals; thick white coating of the tongue; extreme itching. *Worse:* cold water *Better:* rest/quiet, lying down, fresh air	**Antimonium**
Mild case, more like a cold; persistent fever, little itching; but very whiny, clinging, moody; can't stand warmth. *Better:* fresh air, attention, sympathy	**Pulsatilla D12**
Burning itching; restless, wants to scratch constantly; can't lie down or sleep. *Worse:* nights, warm bed	**Rhus toxicodendron D12**
For external use to prevent infection and reduce itch.	**Wecesin powder (Weleda*)**

*Orders filled with prescription.

MEASLES

Measles are also caused by a virus, and infection occurs through the transfer of small drops of moisture. Incubation time is 9 to 15 days. In the first stage, the symptoms are similar to those of a flu, and severe eye complaints are a classic sign. Important for early detection are the small, white spots that appear inside the cheeks in the mouth. Often a high fever sets in that lasts 3 to 5 days. In the second stage, one finds quickly spreading light red spots, starting at the ears and spreading down over the whole body. The spots then merge together, turning into a brownish-red rash. At that point the fever is mild to high. This stage lasts for about 4 to 6 days. Staying inside is essential for recovery. The diagnosis of "measles" must be made by a physician.

KEY SYMPTOMS   **REMEDY**

Stage 1: Symptoms as described above.
Treatment is as for a Viral Infection (Flu).
See page 70.

Stage 2: Slow onset; in a bad mood; persistent,   **Bryonia**
dry cough with stabbing pain; clutches
chest when coughing; lips and mouth
very dry, much thirst, drinks in slow, long
sips; headaches are frequent; constipation.
Worse: motion
Better: drinking, lying down, rest/quiet,
being alone

Classic form with severe eye symptoms;   **Euphrasia**
eyes are red, inflamed, with flow of tears
that is severe and burning, can't stand light;
mild, runny nose, dry cough, sometimes
pounding headaches.
Worse: light, reading, watching TV
Better: rest, lying down in a darkened room

KEY SYMPTOMS	REMEDY
Obvious weakness, terribly exhausted; facial complexion changes between flushed and pale; gets up for a short period of time but must lie down again; eyes are red; dry cough, particularly when lying down.	**Ferrum phosphoricum D12**
Illness proceeds similar to a severe cold that is accompanied by fever; clinging and whining; lids of the eyes are sticky, mild flow of tears; mild runny nose with yellowish-green fluid; lips/mouth dry, but is not very thirsty; dry cough forces the patient to sit up; ear pain. *Worse:* nights, warmth, lying down *Better:* during the day, cool fresh air, attention, sympathy	**Pulsatilla D12**

GERMAN MEASLES

German measles is a highly infectious virus disease. Incubation time is between 14 and 21 days. It usually starts with a slight cold, a runny nose, and swollen neck and throat. A pale red rash appears after approximately 2 days—similar to measles—but it remains distinct and does not merge together. It usually starts behind the ears or on the chest and progresses slowly down to the legs. Temperature is seldom above 100.5° F/38° C. Danger of infecting others is over when the rash begins to subside. German measles usually causes very little discomfort, which makes treatment unnecessary. However, it is important, in case of head, ear, throat, and joint pain, to seek medical attention.

ATTENTION: A German measles infection during the first 3 months of a woman's pregnancy can cause severe complications for her unborn child. Therefore, children who have contracted German measles or could have been infected by the virus must not be allowed to leave their homes—not even for a short shopping trip, where the virus might be allowed to spread.

MUMPS

Mumps are an airborne infecton affecting mostly children. Incubation time is usually 2 to 4 weeks, the first symptoms of swollen salivary glands usually appearing first on one side only, spreading to the other side within 1 or 2 days. Cheeks are swollen, ears stick out, facial features are distorted, and jaws feel tight. Chewing and swallowing becomes painful. Medium to high temperatures. Duration: 4 to 6 days.

IMPORTANT: Seek medical advice and treatment immediately in case of abdominal pain and swelling in the area of the testicles or breasts and ovaries, respectively.

KEY SYMPTOMS	REMEDY
Violent onset with high fever; extremely restless and anxious. For characteristic symptoms/dosages, see Viral Infection (Flu), page 70.	Aconitum D12
Sudden onset on right side with searing, painful glands and high fever. For characteristic symptoms/dosages, see Viral Infection (Flu), page 70.	Belladonna D6
Swollen glands also in the lower jaws; stabbing pain, particularly when swallowing dry (without food; dry mouth, salivating in the morning only; tends toward colds/enlarged tonsils with saliva accumulation.	Barium carbonicum D12
Severe saliva production with much perspiration overthe entire body, saliva constantly dripping from mouth. NOTE: Sometimes symptoms worsen in the initial phase of treatment, with extreme sweating.	Jaborandi D6

KEY SYMPTOMS	REMEDY
Left lymph nodes considerably swollen; severe pain when swallowing, radiating into the left ear; solid food easier to swallow than liquid, but not hot food; doesn't want to be touched or to have anything tight around the neck or body. *Worse:* hot drinks/food, touch, upon awakening *Better:* warmth (external)	**Lachesis D12**
Lymph nodes hard as a stone; throat is raw, dry; has severe pain when swallowing—radiating into the ears; grinds teeth. *Worse:* hot drinks/food, damp cold *Better:* warmth (external), rest/quiet, cold drinks	**Phytolacca D6**
Severe swelling of the ear and saliva glands of the lower jaw; sweet taste in the mouth, heavy flow of saliva. *Worse:* nights, touch, motion *Better:* rubbing, lying on the swollen side	**Plumbum acetum D6**
A mild case, rather like a cold; consistent fever but little pain; still very whiny, clinging; can't tolerate warmth. *Better:* fresh air, attention, sympathy	**Pulsatilla D12**

WHOOPING COUGH

Whooping cough is an airborne bacterial infection whose incubation time is about 7 to 14 days. The first stage of illness is similar to a flu with a cough (catarrh); the fever seldom rises above 102° F/38° C, and it lasts about 1 to 2 weeks. The second stage is marked by the characteristic "whooping" cough, where air is drawn into the lungs with a whistling sound and bronchial mucus is expelled with great difficulty. These symptoms are often accompanied by vomiting and a normal temperature.

Stage 2 lasts for about 6 weeks except in in severe cases, when it can hang on longer. The third stage is marked by a slow decrease in the number of coughing spells, while their duration becomes variable. Often attacks similar to whooping cough occur for many years afterward during very normal colds. Danger of infection is greatest during the first stage, and diagnosis is only possible through a blood test.

Whooping cough is very serious, even life-threatening for babies and children under the age of one year. Any therapy (treatment with antibiotics) must therefore, always and without delay, be conducted by a physician.

Homeopathic remedies can reduce the symptoms and shorten the life of the virus, but remedies must be chosen only by a very experienced lay person. In the absence of such a person, leave the treatment to your physician. IMPORTANT: The characteristics of the cough may sometimes change; if that is the case, reconsider/check the remedy used.

TIP: Whooping cough attacks are not only accompanied by vomiting but also—particularly in the beginning of the second stage—with breathing difficulties, often so extreme that the patient may think he is dying. For that reason, do not let a child sleep alone. In addition, sleep missed during the night should be made up for during the day. Provide a quiet, soothing atmosphere. Give the patient only a light meal in the evening in order to reduce vomiting during the night. Keep the patient in bed as needed.

ATTENTION: Never let sick or infected children come in contact with babies and small children. Keep them indoors for as long as your physician has ordered.

KEY SYMPTOMS   **REMEDY**

Stage 1: Symptoms as described above.
Treatment is as for a Viral Infection (Flu).
See page 70.

KEY SYMPTOMS	REMEDY

Stage 2: Main remedy at the start of second stage when whooping cough becomes evident; coughing attacks, particularly at night, with vomiting; facial complexion pale or bluish, cold sweats; wants to be fanned with cool air; lower legs are cold; nosebleeds; often flatulence.
Worse: warm rooms
Better: cold drinks, fresh air

Carbo vegetabilis D6

Choking, cramp-like cough, particularly when waking up; coughing attacks usually during the night with breathing difficulties; loud rattling noises due to mucus; expelling thick, glassy mucus.
Worse: nights, warmth, warm drinks, motion
Better: cold drinks, cold air

Coccus cacti

Face turns dark red before an attack, gasps for air; afterward short intervals dry, cramp-like coughing; extremely exhausted after coughing attacks, with nosebleeds; very sensitive to cold air.
Worse: nights, cold
Better: warm rooms

Corallium rubrum

Severe, long, cramp-like coughing attacks with breathing difficulties, face turns dark red/blue; vomiting; hands are ice-cold; cramps in arms, legs, and hands while coughing; very exhausted.
Worse: during the night—around 3 A.M.
Better: when sipping water

Cuprum metallicum

Dry, cramp-like coughing, particularly during the night; short, intense attacks of fear of suffocation; face turns dark red to bluish; swelling of the arteries in the head; frequent vomiting and nosebleeds, but not exhausted; clutches chest during coughing spells.
Worse: shortly before midnight

Drosera

KEY SYMPTOMS	REMEDY
Choking; dry, weak coughing with fear of suffocation and mucus rattling in the bronchial tubes; mucus is very thick, almost impossible to evacuate; vomiting, with nosebleeds; cramps; has a pale complexion with dark circles under the eyes. *Worse:* motion *Better:* cold drinks	**Ipecacuanha**
Intense, cramp-like cough with breathing difficulties and fear of dying, particularly during the night; can't exhale—has to be lifted off pillow; face bluish, eyes often red; rattling sounds from the bronchial tubes; attacks less often during the day. Tip: *Mephitis* lasts for only a short time, therefore make sure remedy is given as directed. *Worse:* during the night	**Mephitis**
Remedy of choice when whooping cough has followed measles; dry, cramp-like cough with fear of suffocating when lying down, has to sit up; feels cold easily but can't handle warmth. *Worse:* in the evening, nights, humid/warm weather *Better:* fresh air	**Pulsatilla D12**

Stage 3: For symptoms as stated earlier, *Antimonium.* If further description is needed, see under Bronchial Coughs, page 77–79. Remedies for the second stage of the illness, *Tartaricum, Bryonia,* and *Rumex crispus,* may also be effective for the third stage.

CHAPTER 11

FIRST AID FOR SMALL INJURIES AND WHILE TRAVELING

IMPORTANT TIPS

This chapter is not a substitute for a course in first aid. It deals only with small, everyday complaints and injuries that can be treated with homeopathic remedies. Help for severe injuries—as a matter of course—is subject to the rules of first aid. Therefore, if you have not already done so, take a first aid course at any recommended institutions. They usually also provide first aid courses for children.

At home, as well as when traveling, always be sure you have *Arnica* D12 or the Bach Flower Rescue Remedy. In emergency situations, where immediate medical attention is needed, these remedies have been shown to be very effective: they stabilize both the mental/emotional and physical state of the injured person and are excellent in providing support until medical help arrives. For that reason *Arnica* D12 or the Bach Flower Rescue Remedy belong in every purse, medicine cabinet at home, and first-aid kit in the car.

Directions: Those who are injured and conscious should be given 5 *Arnica* D12 pellets or 5 drops of the rescue remedy every 10 minutes—the latter undiluted directly onto the tongue. For those who are unconscious (or those in shock) the undiluted rescue remedy should be applied several times over the pulse on the inside of the right wrist or rubbed directly into the lips.

ATTENTION: For insurance reasons (third-party responsibility, the possible right to collect damages for pain), always see a physician immediately after an accident and have the type and extent of the injuries recorded. This includes every automobile accident, no matter how minor, and injuries caused by ice on a sidewalk, during athletic and school activities, or a physical attack by a stranger.

Note, especially, the following:

◻ Babies and small children should always be treated by a physician.
◻ If there are lacerations or animal bites, injuries to the head, eyes, breasts, or in the genital or kidney area, always seek medical attention. Until the physician arrives or you get to his office, give *Arnica* D12 or the Bach Flower Rescue Remedy.
◻ If a self-treated wound becomes infected, seek medical treatment immediately.

LACERATIONS, CUTS, AND STAB WOUNDS

Stop bleeding by applying a wet, cold compress; clean and disinfect contaminated wounds with diluted *Calendula* tincture (1 drop of the tincture to 10 drops of water). Choose the appropriate remedy.

Orally: At the onset, take one standard dose every 15 minutes until symptoms improve, then 3 times daily. Externally: Crush a tablet/pellet and either place it directly on a piece of cotton or dissolve it in a half glass of water, saturating a cotton compress with the dilution and applying it to the injury; keep it in place with a bandage, and renew the compress 3 to 5 times daily. ATTENTION: Except for *Calendula*, do not use any of the tinctures for external application.

KEY SYMPTOMS	REMEDY
Injuries caused by nails, thorns, or needles; also those caused by small bites from cats and rodents; stabbing pain and severe red swelling. *Worse:* cold *Better:* warmth	**Apis mellifica**
Main remedy for scrape wounds; usually a salve or compress using a diluted tincture is sufficient; if there are more severe complaints, like a contusion, also take orally.	**Calendula D2**
Main remedy for injuries in areas with nerve tissue, such as fingers, lips, etc.; particularly for cuts and splinters.	**Hypericum**
Like *Apis*, but the injury feels particularly cold. However, the following modalities (though paradoxical) apply: *Worse:* warmth *Better:* cold compresses	**Ledum**
Clean bleeding stab and cut wounds. Especially for sensitive, angry people.	**Staphysagria**

167

CONTUSIONS AND BRUISES

These injuries affect the subcutaneous tissue and the muscles and are the result of a fall or being hit or jammed. Symptoms are painful hematoma and swelling. For eye and nail injuries, also see pages 92 and 114. If there are open wounds, check under Lacerations, page 167.

Apply a cold compress to the injury, or place the injured limb in cold water in order to prevent additional bleeding into the tissues and to relieve pain. Choose the proper homeopathic remedy for internal or external use.

KEY SYMPTOMS	REMEDIES
First-aid remedy for all contusions and bruises; in addition, for very painful injuries that are sensitive to touch as well as black/blue hematomas and all complaints accompanied by severe exhaustion.	**Arnica D12**
Main remedy for injuries in areas of nerve tissue, like fingers, lips, etc.; follow after treatment with *Arnica*.	**Hypericum**
Main remedy for hematoma close to a bone (shin bone, ankle, knee, lower arm, and elbow). Especially for sports injuries; as a follow-up after treatment with *Arnica*.	**Ruta**

SPRAINS AND PULLED LIGAMENTS/MUSCLES

These are usually injuries sustained during sports activities, but also include injuries due to falling on ice, uneven sidewalks, etc. The result is sprained/overstretched ligaments that connect bones, but often muscles are also injured, causing hematoma (see also Contusions and Bruises, page 168). If there is severe pain, rapid and severe swelling, or a dislocated joint or limb, seek medical treatment immediately. Instruction for internal and external application is given under Lacerations, page 167.

KEY SYMPTOMS	REMEDY
First aid for all sprained/pulled ligaments; as additional treatment for very painful swollen tissue that is sensitive to touch and shows black/blue hematoma, as well as all complaints that coincide with severe exhaustion.	**Arnica D12**
Extremely painful, even the slightest movement is unbearable; considerable relief comes from being wrapped tightly; distinct swelling but without hematoma.	**Bryonia**
Swelling with red discoloration and a distinct sense of coldness. *Worse:* warmth *Better:* cold compresses	**Ledum**
Main remedy for joints; despite the pain, can't keep the injured limb still. *Worse:* rest *Better:* warmth	**Rhus toxicodendron**
Hot hematoma close to a bone (shinbone, ankle, ankle, knee, lower arm, or elbow); particularly for sports injuries; also helpful in cases where *Rhus toxicodendron* is not working.	**Ruta**

BURNS AND SUNBURNS

Small first-degree burns, including sunburn, can be self-treated as long as the area burned is not larger than 5 percent of the total skin. Five percent would be equivalent to an area the size of the palm of your hand. However, as soon as blisters begin to develop (as can happen with a second-degree burn) or raw flesh is visible (as with a third-degree), you have an emergency on your hands. Seek medical attention immediately.

General Measures: Hold the very smallest burn or scalding injury close to a heat source for about 5 to 15 seconds (for instance, a candle, range top, oven, or cigarette lighter) until the severe burning pain subsides. No other measure is necessary. Larger burns (first-degree burns) should be covered with a cotton compress that is soaked in a solution of the appropriate remedy (1 standard dose diluted in one half glass of water). The compress should be changed every 15 minutes. In more severe cases, the remedy can also be taken orally; every 15 minutes take one sip of the dilution until symptoms improve, then reduce to 3 times daily.

KEY SYMPTOMS	REMEDY
Sunburn; the skin is shiny/pink and swollen; can't handle warmth.	**Apis mellifica**
Skin is dark red and very sensitive to touch; only to be taken internally.	**Arnica D12**
Skin is light red; there is pounding, pulsating pain.	**Belladonna**
Main remedy for burning pain and sunburn.	**Cantharis**
Painful burning injuries that are healing poorly and for burning scars.	**Causticum**
Sunburn with burning, itching blisters.	**Urtica urens**

IMPORTANT: Do not hold second- and third-degree burn injuries under cold water, and do not remove burned clothing. In cases where clothing has been saturated with an acid-containing chemical, however, it must be removed immediately. In either case, it is an emergency, and until you reach the physician's office or until he reaches you, give the victim *Arnica* tablets/pellets or the Bach Flower Rescue Remedy. If the injured person is conscious, give plenty of water or tea to drink.

HEATSTROKE AND SUNSTROKE

A sunstroke is the result of overexposure to direct sun; the patient has become overheated. The body has absorbed too much heat and is unable to produce perspiration. Sunstroke is generally caused by a lack of fluids and wearing too much clothing (for example, motorcycle garments) in hot weather. Place the victim in the shade or a cool room with the head elevated, and apply a cold, wet cloth to the head and/or body. The following remedies are to be given every 15 minutes; if symptoms do not improve noticeably after 5 standard doses, seek medical attention immediately. IMPORTANT: If the patient has a steadily increasing temperature, stiff neck, shows confusion, or is fainting, call a physician immediately.

KEY SYMPTOMS	REMEDY
Heatstroke; sudden onset of pounding, pulsating pain in the forehead and temples, radiating into the back of the head and neck; face is red, hot, sweaty; pupils are dilated. *Worse:* motion, vibration *Better:* bending head back, slight pressure	**Belladonna D12**
Heatstroke; pounding, almost unbearable pain throughout the head and chest, moving in waves; dizziness; face is red or pale. *Worse:* bending over *Better:* cold compresses for the head, having nosebleeds	**Glonoinum D12**

INSECT BITES

Seek medical attention or go to the emergency room of your local hospital immediately in cases of the following: allergic reaction with restlessness, a dazed feeling, breathing difficulty, and confusion; in cases of known allergies; and for bites in the mouth and throat area. If after one hour of self-treatment, symptoms have not improved, and whenever swelling and pain increases, also seek medical attention immediately.

Remove the stinger with a pair of tweezers and clean and disinfect the wound with a diluted *Calendula* tincture (1 drop of tincture to 10 drops of water). For internal and external application specifications, see page 167.

KEY SYMPTOMS	REMEDY
Stabbing, burning, or itching pain with red shiny swelling; in absence of swelling do not use *Apis*. *Worse:* warmth	**Apis mellifica**
Blood in flesh at bite or sting site (bruise); also when infection has set in.	**Arnica D12**
Main remedy for burning pain that overshadows any other complaint.	**Cantharis**
Main remedy for injuries in nerve-rich areas, like the fingers, lips, etc.; nerves are shooting pain along nerve canals.	**Hypericum**
Itching pain; patient asks for cold compresses; also, if *Apis* did not bring relief after 1 hour; paticularly effective for mosquito and horsefly bites. *Better:* cold	**Ledum**
Persistent pain with blue/red discoloration. ATTENTION: If a red stripe (characteristic of blood poisoning) or swollen lymph nodes develop, seek your physician immediately.	**Lachesis D12***

*Three times daily.

MOTION SICKNESS

Those who have difficulty driving in a car, being on a train, boat, or plane should take the appropriate remedy before leaving. In all other cases, and where no other instructions have been given, take one standard dose of tablets or pellets every 15 minutes until symptoms improve.

KEY SYMPTOMS	REMEDY
Nausea and vomiting during downward motion (as when mountain driving, in car with a soft suspension, on roads alternating between incline and decline, hitting an air pocket when flying); very sensitive to noise, jittery. *Worse:* warm weather, tobacco smoke	**Borax**
Severe dizziness with weak circulation; person is near collapse; must lie down, talks and moves little. *Worse:* sitting up, lack of sleep, eating, thinking about eating *Better:* lying down	**Cocculus**
Extremely sensitive to smell; all odors cause nausea with extreme exhaustion; weak circulatory system with feeling of being cold "inside" to the point of collapse. *Worse:* lack of sleep, motion *Better:* fresh air, moving air, on deck (of boat)	**Colchicum**
Very sick; dizziness with nausea and vomiting; often a weak circulatory system with cold sweat; but can't handle warmth, must open clothing; yellow-green complexion; has to close eyes. *Better:* cool fresh air	**Tabacum**

KEY SYMPTOMS	REMEDY
Same as for *Tabacum*, but with very severe dizziness, nausea, and severe vomiting at the slightest motion and when closing the eyes; extremely sensitive to noise. Particularly for people with seasickness. *Worse:* closing one's eyes *Better:* fixing one's sight on the horizon	**Theridion D12**

TRAVEL ANXIETY AND FEARS

Being slightly nervous before going on a trip is normal. Only when the general well-being and the anticipation of going on a trip is affected by such anxiety should treatment be considered. In cases where a fear is very pronounced, consult with an experienced homeopath. See also Fear, pages 36–38.

KEY SYMPTOMS	REMEDY
Fear of flying and fear of small spaces, standing in line, and crowds; always nervous, irritated, must do everything in a hurry; always expects the worst; also has nervous stomach and intestinal problems with cramps and diarrhea.	**Argentum nitricum D12***
Travel sickness: growing restlessness, constant urge to urinate, diarrhea, headaches, heart problems, jittery, signs of paralysis, insomnia. Especially for cautious and shy people.	**Gelsemium D12**

*In acute anxiety attacks, 1 dose every 15 minutes until improvement; no more than 5 doses.

CHAPTER 12

BEFORE AND AFTER SURGERY

PREPARING FOR SURGERY

Not only are homeopathic remedies able to treat already existing complaints, but they are also able to prevent symptoms from developing in the first place. This makes them an ideal preparation for regular as well as oral surgeries. If a patient has a greater likelihood of having excessive bleeding and/or thrombosis, the choice of the remedy should be left to an experienced physician or homeopath. Also, the surgeon needs to be informed about what kind of remedy has been taken.

KEY SYMPTOMS	REMEDY
Main remedies to counteract the physical, emotional, and mental trauma of surgery.	**Arnica C6** and **D12**

Instruction: Shortly before and after surgery, take 1 standard dose each of C6; then, depending on the severity of the pain, 1 standard dose of D12, 1 to 3 times daily.

POST-OPERATIVE CARE

Here, homeopathy is trying to support the healing process, as well as to prevent possible complications.

KEY SYMPTOMS	REMEDY
After-affects of anesthesia: nausea, feeling dazed, dizziness; directly after complaints have set in and after they have lessened; pellets are the best.	**Nux vomica D6**
After the after-affects of the anesthesia have subsided for the relief of the physical as well as the mental/emotional trauma of the operation; for the prevention of bleeding.	**Arnica D12***

*One standard dose 1 to 3 times daily.

KEY SYMPTOMS	REMEDY
Severely painful wounds; feeling bruised; sometimes pain improves with light movement; particularly for scarring after abdominal surgery: here, give one standard dose 3 times daily for several weeks.	**Bellis perennis D6**
After intestinal surgery and after the removal of hemorrhoids.	**Collinsonia**
Painful wounds after surgery in areas of nerve-rich tissue, after injury to a nurve, and also after an amputation.	**Hypericum**
Painful wounds after clean incisions, particularly cuts in the abdominal area; after the removal of kidney stones. For patients who feel as if their personal boundaries have been violated.	**Staphysagria**
After eye surgery, particularly after the the implantation of an artificial lens.	**Senega**
After eye surgery resulting in severe sensitivity to light and vision problems.	**Zincum metallicum**

CARE AFTER BONE FRACTURE

KEY SYMPTOMS	REMEDY
Main remedy after a fracture, take until everything has healed.	**Symphytum D6***
Bone fracture with injury to the periosteum; irritating pain or a feeling as if the bone is being "scraped."	**Acidum phosphoricum D6***
Bone fractures that are healing poorly. Especially for people who have "fine" bones, most of all children, and in the presence of osteoporosis.	**Calcarea phosphorica D6***

*Until healing is complete, one standard dose 3 times daily (for about 2 months).

CHAPTER 13

THE HOMEOPATHIC HOME MEDICINE CHEST

A MEDICINE CHEST FOR BEGINNERS

Since a beginner should only treat small, uncomplicated problems, only a small basic supply of homeopathic remedies is needed. The choice of how to use them is left to the individual—more or less. With children in the house, the recommendation is to use only pellets, tablets, powders, or lotions, since these do not contain alcohol.

Have the following on hand:

Aconitum D12
Apis mellifica D6
Arnica D12
Arsenicum album D12
Belladonna D6
Bryonia D6
Cantharis D6
Cepa D6
Chamomilla D12
Gelsemium D12
Hypericum D6
Ledum D6
Nux vomica D12
Pulsatilla D12

In addition, have a *Calendula* salve (like *Calendumed* DHU) on hand.

A MEDICINE CHEST FOR
EXPERIENCED LAY PERSONS

For those who already have experience in the use of homeopathic self-treatment and feel sure that they can treat more complicated problems, the following remedies should be on hand:

Causticum D6
Dulcamara D6
Euphrasia D6
Ferrum phosphoricum D6
Hepar sulfuris D6
Ignatia D12
Lachesis D12
Natrum chloratum D12
Rhus toxicodendron D12
Ruta D6
Silicea D12
Sulfur D6

In addition to these basic remedies, stock your medicine cabinet with all those that your homeopath has prescribed, as well as those most frequently used in your household. For instance, if you frequently experience stomach problems of the type *Antimonium crudum* or kidney problems of the type *Berberis*, you obviously should have those remedies on hand.

PROPER STORAGE OF REMEDIES

Stored properly, homeopathic remedies have a virtually limitless shelf life. However, proper storage means—first and foremost—protection from light (storing them in dark glass bottles), keeping them cool and dry, and placing them as far away as possible from any source of electricity, including TV and radio. This means that bathrooms and kitchens are not appropriate places to keep these medications. The best place is a bedroom, as long as it is kept cool.

Excessive heat can damage the remedies, so it is also a good practice not to keep your medicine travel kit in the car when the weather is hot. And the importance of keeping homeopathic remedies out of the reach of children goes without saying.

PART III

THE HOMEOPATHIC
MATERIA MEDICA

How to use this Materia Medica, a listing of
the characteristics of each remedy

No patient and no illness shows all the symptoms listed in the Materia Medica. Take, for instance, an inflamed throat; it is important only that the actual complaints correspond with the symptoms and the modalities of the remedy. Do, however, read the total list of symptoms. Experience has shown that additional symptoms are found—like a specific mental/emotional condition ("very clinging," or "wants to be left alone") or sleeping in a certain position ("sleeps with the hands over the head")—which will help to confirm the choice of remedy. In addition, this is one way of learning more about the most important remedies used for self-treatment and their usefulness for other complaints.

The modalities given at the end of many of the descriptions—"*Worse*" and "*Better*"—are applicable to all symptoms listed. Where they deviate and are applicable only to an individual symptom, "*W*" or "*B*" follows immediately after that particular symptom. If a single symptom is followed by a comma, then the modality "*W*" or "*B*" refers to that symptom only. If a modality refers to several symptoms, they are separated by a semicolon or period. Used in the following entries, for instance:

Nosebleeds; pain as if from a band tied around the head, *W:* pressure, noise (*meaning that only the pain gets worse with pressure or noise, not the nosebleeds*).

Throat dry and sore; difficulty swallowing. *B:* warm food (*meaning the dryness and the soreness in the throat and the difficulty swallowing improve when eating warm food*).

ACIDUM PHOSPHORICUM

An important remedy for mental/emotional exhaustion, specifically when due to worry; also for school-age children who have experienced recent growth spurts; as well as after severe illness and infection.

CHARACTERISTIC SYMPTOMS

Mental/Emotional: Very sad, desperate after worry and emotional shock; does not want to be talked to. Tired, exhausted due to the loss of body fluids or rapid growth; listless, indifferent, can't concentrate, forgetful, slow-witted.

Head: Intense pain in the center of the head and at both temples. Headaches due to eyestrain or after sex. Premature graying, loss of hair. A pale complexion with circles under the eyes.

Sensory Organs: Sunken eyes, glassy; pupils dilated. Nose itching, pokes nose; nose bleeds. Lips are dry and cracked. Tongue is swollen, dry. Bites tongue during sleep.

Breathing Organs: Weak feeling in the chest after speaking. Pressure behind the chest bone hinders breathing. Dry, itching, irritated cough. Heart palpitation after worry and during rapid growth spurts in children.

Digestion: Prefers juicy liquids and cold milk. Does not feel good and is nauseated after sour food. Visibly distended abdomen with loud rumbling and pain in the navel area. Painless, whitish, watery diarrhea with a lot of gas; does not seem to diminish energy; sometimes incontinent.

Urinary Tract: Plenty of urine, milky. Increased urge to urinate during the night.

Extremities/Back: Very weak extremities, particularly arms and legs. Cramps and tearing pain in the extremities during the night. Feels as if the bones are being "scraped." Itching between the fingers and in their joints.

Skin: Bad complexion, acne, an urticaria rash with burning and tingling.

Worse: During the night, with cold, exertion, excitement, and receiving attention.

Better: For warmth and sleeping.

PROVEN INDICATORS FOR ACIDUM PHOSPHORICUM

Sadness, depression, mental and concentration difficulties, loss of hair, bad skin, headaches, digestive problems, aching joints, and feeling tired.

ACONITUM

Aconitum is the main remedy for the early stages of illnesses caused by cold weather, cold drafts, or fright and shock. Symptoms appear suddenly and forcefully. Unbearable pain with restlessness, often fear of death. In the absence of restlessness and fear, Aconitum is not the proper remedy.

CHARACTERISTIC SYMPTOMS

Mental/Emotional: Frequent attacks of fear of death, including in nightmares. Also fears crowds of people.

Head: Pounding headache, dizziness, nausea when getting up. When lying down, one cheek is flushed, and the other is pale, or both are flushed, and both are pale when getting up. One-sided pain in facial nerves radiating into the jaw and teeth.

Sensory Organs: Eyelids are inflamed and swollen; heavy tearing, very sensitive to light. Earaches; external part of the ear is hot, swollen, and red; very sensitive to noise. Nose stuffed up; extreme sensitivity to smell; nosebleeds with light red blood.

Breathing Organs: Throat is red and dry; has a hoarse, dry, croaking cough; stabbing pain in the chest; feeling as if there is a stone lying on the chest; breathing difficulties with fear of having a coronary, heart is racing, blood pressure elevated. *W:* during the night and after midnight.

Digestion: Vomiting with profuse sweating, thirsty for a lot of cold water. Bloody hemorrhoids, stabbing pain. Foul-smelling stool, green in color and spinach-like consistency.

Urinary Tract: Urine is scant, hot, and urination is painful, but sometimes also liberal with diarrhea and sweating. Holding urination back causes pain and restlessness.

Extremities: Hands are hot, feet cold; numb, tingling, stabbing pain. Joints are painful, swollen, numb; any kind of movement worsens condition.

Skin: Dry, hot, can't stand warmth.

Worse: In the evening, nights, warmth. Lying on left side, at touch.

Better: Fresh, cool air, rest, sweating.

PROVEN INDICATORS FOR ACONITUM

Fear, panic attacks, fright/shock (also after an accident, surgery), insomnia, a cold in the beginning stages with shivering, tonsillitis, conjunctivitis, ear-, head-, and toothaches; neuralgia, cystitis, early stages of chicken pox, measles, whooping cough, and mumps.

ALUMINA

Important characteristics are dry skin, also dry mucus membranes, either muscle weakness or tension, as well as worsening of the symptoms in the morning. Especially for these symptoms in old people.

CHARACTERISTIC SYMPTOMS

Mental/Emotional: Anxious, moody, forgetful, depressed in the morning, B: during the course of the day. Always in a hurry. Time seems to go slowly.
Head: Dizziness.
Sensory Organs: Burning, itching eyelids that stick together. Nose rough, cracked, and stuffed up. Mouth either dry or has an increased flow of saliva. Teeth ache when chewing.
Breathing Organs: Throat is dry and rough; has difficulty swallowing, B: warm food. Feels as if a lump is stuck in the throat.
Digestion: Strange urges. An aversion against meat. Eats only small bites. Intestinal movement slow, even soft stool is excreted slowly. Passing stool normal, but hard and dry; bleeds when passing stool.
Urinary Tract: Has to press, as when passing stool.
Female Genitalia: much watery-sharp discharge. Menstruation too early, scant, short, but weakening.
Extremities: Arms and legs heavy, weak, "going to sleep" easily. Trips when walking. Nails brittle, sensation of splinters stuck under the nails.
Skin: Dry, wrinkled; mucus membranes dried out. Unbearable itching in warm bed.
Worse: In the morning, afternoons, because of warmth in bed, from walking, and from the smallest amount of alcohol.
Better: In the evening, for fresh air, and moderate movement.

PROVEN INDICATORS FOR ALUMINA

Insomnia, lazy intestines/constipation, brittle nails, problems during menstruation, dryness and itching of the vagina.

ANTIMONIUM CRUDUM

This is an important stomach remedy, particularly for small children and older people, often in the presence of weight problems. Central symptoms are irritability and a thick, white coating of the tongue.

CHARACTERISTIC SYMPTOMS

Mental/Emotional: Irritability, nothing is right, moody, sour or sad, depressed; children don't want to be touched or looked at.

Head: Has headaches after too much sour food (has headaches particularly from wine, sweets, and sun).

Sensory Organs: Skin at the entrance to the nose, on the upper lip, and at the corners of the mouth is cracked. Thick, white coating of the tongue.

Breathing Organs: Hoarseness with loss of voice. Coughing is worse in warm rooms, has an itching chest.

Digestion: Lack of appetite, but an urge for sweet and sour food. Nausea, burping, heartburn, abdomen visibly distended after a meal; slimy-watery diarrhea with lumps after sour food, sweet baked goods, and bread.

Extremities: Calluses and painful, inflamed corns. Brittle nails.

Skin: Dry itching in warm bed. Dermatitis, like measles or blisters. Warts.

Worse: In the evening, for sour food, wine, heat, water, cold baths and compresses.

Better: For being outdoors, warm humid air, and rest.

PROVEN INDICATORS FOR ANTIMONIUM CRUDUM

Contact dermatitis, intolerance to food, nervous stomach, hangover headaches, corns, calluses, brittle nails, and chicken pox.

ANTIMONIUM TARTARICUM

A proven remedy for coughs, particularly for a bronchial cough with rattling sounds but little expectoration, great weakness, and exhaustion.

CHARACTERISTIC SYMPTOMS

Mental/Emotional: Very depressed, does not want to be alone.

Head: Pale, hollow complexion, cold sweat. Dull pain in forehead as if "squeezed" in vise, W: closing eyes and sleeping. Dizziness. Chin and lower jaw jittery.

Sensory Organs: Paste-like, white, thick coating of the tongue, edges are red.

Breathing Organs: Rattling cough with a sense of suffocation, a lot of tough, white mucus that is difficult to cough up; severe exhaustion; breathing difficulty.

Digestion: Nausea, vomiting, with anxiety and exhaustion, mainly after meals. Desire for sour food, especially apples and fruit. Sips a lot of cold water.

Extremities: General weakness.

Sleep: Very sleepy and dazed.

Worse: Evenings, during night (3 A.M.), when lying down, and humid/warm rooms.

Better: Sitting up, after burping, coughing up mucus, and vomiting.

PROVEN INDICATORS FOR ANTIMONIUM TARTARICUM
Bronchial cough, complains of sour stomach.

APIS MELLIFICA

This remedy is for complaints that are similar to the result of a bee sting. Important symptoms are a feeling of tightness, stabbing pain, edemas, and fever without being thirsty.

CHARACTERISTIC SYMPTOMS
Mental/Emotional: Clumsy, restless, whiny, can't concentrate.

Head: Dull ache in the back of head, as if having been hit; head is flushed and hot, with dizziness. Face is swollen and red, or wax-like and pale.

Sensory Organs: Eyelids are swollen, red, and hot; tears are hot and burning; eyes are sensitive to light. Sudden stabbing pain in the eyes. Nose is swollen, red, and inflamed. Mouth and tongue are fiery red, look shiny, swollen, sore with blisters, as if burned. Gums and upper lip are swollen.

Breathing Organs: Throat is shiny red, glossy, and swollen; tonsils are red and swollen. Throat feels constricted, swollen inside and out, pain is sharp as if stuck by a fishbone. Hoarseness. Coughs, difficulty breathing. *W:* lying down, sleeping.

Digestion: Stomach feels sore; no thirst.

Urinary Tract: Urine is sparse, intensely yellow; has burning, stabbing pain when urinating, particularly during the very last drops.

Extremities: Fluid accumulation in ankles and feet. Knees are swollen with the skin shiny; stabbing pain.

Skin: Very sensitive, stabbing pain. Sudden swelling of the whole body.

Worse: Heat in any form, for touch, late in the afternoon, and after having slept on the right side.

Better: For fresh air, cold baths, and when not covered.

PROVEN INDICATORS FOR APIS MELLIFICA
Throat, tonsil, and gum inflammation and conjunctivitis, cystitis, rash, stabbing and splinter injuries, insect bites, sunburn, and fevers without thirst.

ARGENTUM NITRICUM

"Anxiously waiting" is the key symptom of this remedy. It is able to heal a variety of complaints, especially those due to nerves.

CHARACTERISTIC SYMPTOMS

Mental/Emotional: Anxious, nervous, restless, melancholy, and impulsive. Is always in a hurry. Time passes too slowly. Strange impulses.

Head: Dull pain, *B:* pressure. Pounding tension headaches. Also migraine headaches due to emotional tension, often with weakness, jitters, and dizziness with ear humming. Sensitive scalp. Facial neuralgia. Pale, hollow complexion.

Sensory Organs: Vision impaired, specks in front of the eyes, hazy vision; can't handle light in warm rooms. Mouth is very sensitive to cold. Has toothaches after cold or sour food. Bleeding gums.

Breathing Organs: Forced to clear throat due to too much mucus. Feeling as if there is a splinter stuck in the throat.

Chest: Hoarseness, breathing difficulty. *W:* tobacco smoke.

Heart: Pounding heart, *W:* lying on the right side.

Digestion: Great desire for something sweet. Many stomach problems with annoying burping, *B:* after burping. Pit of stomach painfully swollen. Visibly distended abdomen. Watery, greenish diarrhea with flatulence and a consistency like spinach, *W:* excitement.

Urinary Tract: Incontinence.

Unstable gait. Lower legs stiff and weak.

Worse: Warmth in any form, at night, for eating cold food, after eating, and from excitement.

Better: For cold, fresh air, pressure, and burping.

PROVEN INDICATORS FOR ARGENTUM NITRICUM

Stage fright, test fright, travel nerves, fear of height and flying, agoraphobia, headaches, migraine, and nervous stomach and intestines.

ARNICA

Absolutely essential for physical injuries due to falls, hits, and bruises. But *Arnica* is also helpful in cases of emotional hurts. The most important identifying symptom is the sense of being exhausted.

CHARACTERISTIC SYMPTOMS

Mental/Emotional: Wants to be alone; won't talk about complaints, says everything is okay. Nervous, overly sensitive, moody. Agoraphobia.

Head: Hot, but body is cold. Dizziness at the slightest movement.

Sensory Organs: Overly tired eyes after TV watching and close-up work; bad breath, like rotten eggs. Dark red nosebleeds after coughing.

Breathing Organs: Severe, cramp-like, dry coughs after a whooping cough; can't cough up mucus. W: exertion, chest pain radiating into the arms.

Digestion: Loss of appetite. Desire for vinegar. Foul-smelling burping with nausea and vomiting. Cramp-like pain, as if the stomach is being pressed against the spine. Heavy, foul-smelling, brown diarrhea.

Extremities: The whole body feels as if beaten up or squashed. Even the bed is too hard. Great fear of being touched and approached.

Skin: The hematoma is blue to black. Small boils.

Sleep: Restless, can't sleep in spite of being overtired. Nightmares.

Worse: In the evening, at night, for touch, movement, and in a hard bed.

Better: For rest and lying down.

PROVEN INDICATORS FOR ARNICA

Contusions, bruises, agoraphobia, emotional shock, insomnia, tiredness, exhaustion, fatigue, burns, sunburns, before and after surgery, dental procedures, and giving birth.

ARSENICUM ALBUM

Central symptoms are severe exhaustion with shivering after the slightest exertion and burning pain that—except for headaches—improve with warmth. There is also extreme fear and restlessness, and all complaints get worse during the night. Particularly for stomach and intestinal problems and the aftermath of a shock.

CHARACTERISTIC SYMPTOMS

Mental/Emotional: Extreme fear, including fear of death, that can cause breaking into cold sweat and physical restlessness. Can't stand to be alone.

Head: Headache, B: cold compresses. Dandruff, hair loss. Hollow face, spotty, red. Cracked lips that burn.

Sensory Organs: Inflamed, swollen eyes with burning tears, also dry eyes; very light-sensitive. Nose stuffed, but drips thin, watery slime; sneezing attacks. Tongue dry, clear, and red. Gums bleed; a sense that teeth are too long.

Breathing Organs: Throat is swollen, constricted, can hardly swallow, has burning pain. Dry cough with breathing difficulty, little mucus is coughed up, W: midnight. Burning chest pain on the right side, B: when getting up.
Heart: Pulse quickens at the slightest movement.
Digestion: Burning pain with a great thirst for cold water; drinks it in big gulps. Nausea and vomiting after eating. Has an aversion to fruit, vegetables, ice cream, and sour food. Fear "sits" in the stomach. A thin, watery, burning stool, particularly after eating and during the night. Burning hemorrhoids.
Female Genitalia: Heavy, thick, yellow discharge. Menstruation coming on too early and heavy.
Extremities: Jittery, weak, heavy, has cramps in calf, muscle twitches.
Skin: Dry, rough, scaly, and burning itches.
Sleep: Restless and anxious. Grinds teeth, has attacks of suffocation, sleeps with hands over the head, and needs a lot of pillows.
Worse: After midnight, cold and humid weather, at the seashore, movement.
Better: For heat and cold drinks.

PROVEN INDICATORS FOR ARSENICUM ALBUM

Anxious feelings, panic attacks, disturbed sleep, stomach and intestinal infections, headaches, migraine, body aches, tiredness, palpitations, fever, loss of hair.

BELLADONNA

Belladonna is the main remedy for the early stages of suddenly appearing complaints with pounding, pulsating pain and severe redness of the skin. It is especially characterized by a fever with no thirst.

CHARACTERISTIC SYMPTOMS

Mental/Emotional: All senses are overreacting, and any outside stimuli is too much. Lives in his own world, ignores surroundings.
Head: Pounding pain, particularly at the temples, forehead, and back of the head, W: lying down, chewing, light, noise, in the afternoon. B: pressure. Dizziness from tilting to the left or backwards. Face is intensely red and hot. Facial neuralgia with muscle twitching.
Sensory Organs: Eyes are rigid and shiny; pupils are dilated. The conjunctiva is red and dry with burning pain. Can't tolerate light. Frequent nosebleeds and has a heightened sense of smell. Extreme, throbbing ear pain,

often with a fever. Mouth and lips are dry. Tongue is the color of bright strawberries. Tooth abscesses.

Breathing Organs: Throat is red and dry, as if glazed, particularly on the right side. Feels as if bound up; has difficulty swallowing. Very painful larynx. Dry, irritating cough, W: nights.

Female Breasts: Throbbing pain, breasts are red, heavy, and very painful. Red strips radiating out from the nipples.

Heart: Heart pounds rapidly at the slightest exertion.

Digestion: Loss of appetite. Extreme thirst for cold water. Abdomen distended, hot, and can't tolerate touch. Stool is thin and greenish. Hemorrhoids.

Urinary Tract: Frequent urges to urinate; urine sufficient, but flow also suppressed in cases of acute cystitis.

Female Genitalia: Vagina hot and dry. Menstruation is too early, bright red, hot, and severely painful with a sense of "pulling down."

Extremities: Cold hands and feet.

Skin: Hot, dry, and swollen scarlet red. In case of a fever, there is steaming heat from the portion of the body that is under the covers, but the person still wants to stay covered; feet are ice-cold.

Sleep: Restless. Grinds teeth.

Worse: In the evening, lying down, to touch, noise, vibration, and drafts.

Better: In partially upright position, at rest, pressure, stretching, and fresh air.

PROVEN INDICATORS FOR BELLADONNA

At the beginning of a cold or a throat, larynx, tonsil, sinus, or conjunctiva infection; earaches and toothaches, gingivitis, abscesses, sore skin, cystitis, painful kidneys, mastitis, menstruation problems, the early stages of chicken pox, measles, mumps, whooping cough, burns, sunburns, and sunstroke.

BRYONIA

The central symptoms for this remedy are intense irritability, stabbing, irritating pain, dry, soft tissues, and physical weakness. Complaints develop slowly, and everything gets worse with motion.

CHARACTERISTIC SYMPTOMS

Mental/Emotional: Extreme irritability, moody, wants to be left alone. Anxious, and gets anxious quickly. For children who don't want to be carried.

Head: Burning pain, particularly on the right, W: moving the eyes.

Headaches in the forehead, where there is sinus infection. Nausea and dizziness when getting up, and especially in warm rooms. The face is a pale, yellowish color, swollen and bloated. The hair is very greasy.

Sensory Organs: Frequent nosebleeds before menstruation; also in the morning, which relieves headaches. Cold with shooting pain in the forehead. Ear noises. Lips are like parchment paper, dry, and cracked. Mouth and tongue are dry. Yellow-brown or dark brown coating of the tongue; where there is an upset stomach, the coating is thick and white. A foul, bitter taste in the mouth.

Breathing Organs: Dry with stabbing pain when swallowing. Has a thick mucus that is difficult to cough up. A dry, hacking cough, during which the person clutches the chest, W: entering a warm room, eating, drinking. B: sitting upright or lying on the painful side.

Female Breasts: Sensitive, hot, hard. Pulling pain at the middle of the cycle.

Digestion: Very thirsty for cold water, drinks in small sips. Nauseous, weak, and dizzy when getting up. Vomits after drinking and eating warm food. Feels as if there is a stone in the stomach. Very sensitive to touch. W: for taking deep breaths, coughing, and pressure. Constipation; stool is hard, dark, crumbly; but also diarrhea due to heat or cold drinks.

Female Genitalia: Menstruation too early, too heavy. Painful right ovary.

Male Genitalia: Stabbing pain in the prostate.

Extremities/Back: Joints red, swollen; has hot, stabbing pain also in the neck and spine.

Worse: In the morning, for warmth, hot weather, motion, touch, and sitting upright.

Better: When lying down on the painful side, for pressure, rest, quietness, and cold in any form.

PROVEN INDICATORS FOR BRYONIA

Irritability, headaches, migraines, insomnia, a bronchial cough, stomach and intestinal problems, nervous stomach, toothaches, mastitis, menstruation problems, measles, sprains, and pulled ligaments.

CALCAREA CARBONICA

Calcarea carbonica is an excellent remedy for constitution therapy but is also very helpful to treat weakness that is a leftover from a previous illness or overwork. It is especially useful for blond and more or less lethargic people who tend to be overweight.

CHARACTERISTIC SYMPTOMS

Mental/Emotional: A variety of fears: of accidents, illness, and going insane. Forgetful, can't concentrate, is thick-headed. Has an aversion to exertion in any form.

Head: Headaches after mental work or strain, while hands and feet are ice-cold. B: for sneezing. Right side of the head is ice-cold. Heavy perspiration of the head during the night. Hair loss.

Sensory Organs: Eyes get tired easily and are sensitive to light, showing increased tearing in the morning and outdoors. Nose is dry, sore, and ulcerous. Nose polyps. Gets cold when weather changes. Ears are sensitive to cold and make cracking noises; they are often infected because of the swelling of the lymph nodes. Impaired hearing. A sour taste in the mouth, and the tongue is dry during the night. The tip of it burns. Gums bleed. The teeth are sensitive. Cavities.

Breathing Organs: The tonsils are swollen frequently, infected. Stabbing pain when swallowing. Morning hoarseness without pain. Difficulty breathing during exertion (climbing stairs). Tickling cough during the night. Breasts are very touch and pressure sensitive.

Digestion: Heartburn with loud burping. Hiccups with sour vomiting. Stomach cramps. Desire for eggs, salt, and sweets. An aversion to milk and fat. Loses appetite after overworking. Can't handle anything tight around the waist. Large, hard, whitish stool or diarrhea, passing undigested food. Burning hemorrhoids and anal prolapse.

Male Genitalia: Premature ejaculation.

Female Genitalia: Burning itching in the vagina, milky-white discharge. Swollen, sensitive breasts before menstruation. Period is too early, too heavy with dizziness, toothaches, and damp/cold feet.

Extremities: Feet damp/cold, the soles of feet are rough. Cramps in the calf. Brittle nails.

Skin: Limp and pale. Problem with wounds healing. Allergic dermatitis.

Fever: Night sweats, particularly the head, neck, breasts. Fever in the afternoon with heavy perspiration and stomach problems.

Worse: In the evening, at night, for exertion, from cold dampness in any from, from standing, and from being alone.

Better: For dry weather, lying down on the painful side, and sneezing.

PROVEN INDICATORS FOR CALCAREA CARBONICA

Fear, tiredness, depression, exhaustion, insomnia, migraines, flatulence, a feeling of fullness, bad skin, nettle fever, sore skin, brittle nails, hair loss, teething problems, premenstrual problems, and complaints during menopause.

IMPORTANT: *Calcarea carbonica* does not go together with *Bryonia*. Do not take these remedies in succession. Also, *Sulfur* is not used after a treatment with *Calcarea carbonica*.

CALCAREA PHOSPHORICA

This remedy is similar to *Calcarea carbonica* but is used more often when the tissues are affected as well as bones. It is also used for pale, anemic, fragile, dissatisfied, and restless children with a weak digestive system and cold hands and feet, especially during puberty.

CHARACTERISTIC SYMPTOMS
Mental/Emotional: Moody, forgetful, dissatisfied. Always ready to jump.
Head: Headaches with flatulence in school-age children, W: for changes in the weather and mental work.
Teeth: Slow tooth development, then quick loss due to cavities.
Breathing Organs: Tonsils swollen; opening the mouth is painful. Polyps.
Digestion: Frequent vomiting, frequent flatulence, B: burping. Desire for salty, smoked meat. Very hungry and thirsty. Stomach cramps when trying to eat. Abdominal surface limp and caved in. Diarrhea—particularly during teething—is greenish-white with foul-smelling gas; but also has hard stool with bleeding.
Extremities/Back: Cold, numb, stiff, and painful. Falls asleep easily. Has bone and joint pain; shows delayed healing after injuries.
Worse: For damp/cold weather and changes in the weather.
Better: For warm, dry weather, in the summer, and for eating.

PROVEN INDICATORS FOR CALCAREA PHOSPHORICA
Headaches, tiredness, exhaustion, fatigue, overwork, sensitivity to weather, cavities, bone injuries, and growing pains.

CALENDULA

Calendula is an absolutely essential remedy for treating local infections, supporting wound healing, and relieving pain after injuries, particularly cuts, scrapes, tears, and burn wounds. It can also be helpful after tooth extraction. Best in the form of a salve (for example, *Calendumed* from DHU) or as a compress from a diluted tincture.

195

CARBO VEGETABILIS

The central symptoms of this remedy are twofold: the first is a physical and mental/emotional slowdown that often appears after a previous illness; the second is a series of digestive problems. *Carbo vegetabilis* is an especially appropriate remedy for lethargic people who have a tendency to be overweight.

CHARACTERISTIC SYMPTOMS
Mental/Emotional: Anxious, with fear of the dark. Lethargic and unmotivated. Shows a sudden loss of memory.

Head: Headaches after overeating. Scalp itches from warmth in bed; hair loss. Head feels heavy, a hat feels like a "weight." Complexion is pale, even during exertion; face is distended, cold, and sweaty.

Sensory Organs: Nosebleeds in the morning; also nosebleeds during exertion; the tip of the nose is scaly and red. A whitish-brown or yellow-brown coating of the tongue. Gums bleeding during the brushing of teeth; periodontosis.

Breathing Organs: Hoarseness with loss of voice, W: for speaking and in the evening. Tickling sensation in the larynx. Coughing with burning sensation in the chest. Mucus rattles with a sense of suffocation, W: in the evening, after eating and speaking. B: for fresh air.

Digestion: Hungry with a feeling of weakness, but eating brings no relief. Stomach cramps radiate into the chest, ½ to 1 hour after eating. Sour burps and a visible distended abdomen with foul-smelling gas, especially seen in nursing mothers. B: burping, releasing gas. Can't handle anything tight around the waist.

Extremities: Heavy, has difficulty falling asleep. Lower legs and feet are cold. Cramps in the soles of the feet. Red, swollen frostbite on the toes.

Worse: In the evening, at night, for cold, greasy food, butter, coffee, milk, wine, in humid/warm weather, and in warm rooms.

Better: For fresh air and burping.

PROVEN INDICATORS FOR CARBO VEGETABILIS
Tiredness, exhaustion, fatigue, difficulty with concentration and memory after illness, stomach and intestinal problems, heartburn, flatulence, hair loss, varicose veins, and whooping cough.

CAULOPHYLLUM

Caulophyllum is an important remedy in the preparation for a birth and for healing menstrual problems. The mental/emotional situation is similar to that of *Ignatia*.

CHARACTERISTIC SYMPTOMS
Mental/Emotional: Moody, fearful. Very irritable, tense, restless, has sleeping problems, is whiny. Wants to be left alone.
Head: Headaches, during menstruation and especially on the left side, W: bending down. Face is pale and damp.
Digestion: Vomiting during menstruation.
Menstruation: Too early, too late, or spare; very sensitive to cold. Contraction-like pain radiates into the thighs, lower legs, feet, and toes.
Uterus: Muscles and ligaments are weak, dropping all the way to collapse. Discharge causes soreness. Weak contraction. Postnatal contraction radiates to the groin area.
Extremities/Back: Rheumatic pain in the small joints (fingers, wrists, toes, and ankles). Sensitive spine and stiffness in the back.
Worse: At night, for cold, and for loud noise.
Better: For warmth, quiet, and being alone.

PROVEN INDICATORS FOR CAULOPHYLLUM
Menstrual problems, preparation for birth, and exhaustion after giving birth. IMPORTANT: *Caulophyllum* does not combine well with *Coffea*; do not give these remedies in succession.

CAUSTICUM

A very important remedy used in constitution therapies, *Causticum* is also helpful for acute problems that are combined with burns, roughness, and soreness of the skin, and after emotional stress.

CHARACTERISTIC SYMPTOMS
Mental/Emotional: Nervous and insecure. Sad, depressed, melancholy, hopeless. Cries quickly. Very empathetic. Fears large animals.
Head: Pain in the left side of the forehead. Facial neuralgia due to cold air.
Sensory Organs: Upper lids are heavy, and eyes close involuntarily. Lower

lids are weak, as if paralyzed, particularly during a cold. Feeling as if there is sand in the eyes. There is noise and a sense of echo in the ears. Has a dry cold, with severe sneezing attacks, and a stuffed-up nose. Tongue is heavy. The gums bleed.

Breathing Organs: Paralyzed vocal cords. Hoarseness, particularly in the morning and evening. Thick mucus, almost impossible to cough up, is much more likely to be swallowed. Coughing with incontinence, *W:* warm bed, *B:* cold water in small sips.

Digestion: Frequent, sudden, stabbing pain in the rectum; unsuccessful urges to pass stool, passing stool is easier while standing. Burning hemorrhoids.

Urinary Tract: Bed-wetting in children right after they go to sleep. Incontinence when coughing, sneezing, laughing, and during sleep. Holding back urination after giving birth or having surgery.

Extremities/Back: Restless legs during the night. Muscle twitches. Weak muscles and ankles, unsteady gate. Tearing pain in the joint. *B:* in a warm bed and for stretching.

Skin: Warts, particularly at the tip of the finger and on the nose. Skin folds are sore and also between the thighs. Healing after burn injuries is interrupted, and scars break open again. Diaper rash during teething.

Worse: In the afternoon, at night, for cold, dry wind, and dry/hot weather.

Better: For cold drinks, humid weather, and a warm wrap.

PROVEN INDICATORS FOR CAUSTICUM

Sadness, depression, fear of large animals, hoarseness, corns, warts, problems with wounds healing, and sore skin. IMPORTANT: *Causticum* does not go together well with *Phosphorus*; do not use these remedies in succession.

CEPA
(formerly called Allium cepa)

This is an important remedy for treating a cold, particularly in cases where there are eye, nose, and throat complaints. The complaints usually start on the left and then wander over to the right side.

CHARACTERISTIC SYMPTOMS

Mental/Emotional: The eyes are very sensitive to light, which increases tear development; the discharge is mild. Nose burns, with an acid-like, watery discharge making the nose and upper lip sore. Severe sneezing attacks.

Sensory Organs: Ticklish, painful coughing attacks, whooping cough in the early stages with vomiting and flatulence.

Urinary Tract: Frequent urges with burning when urinating.

Extremities: Stabbing nerve pain after injuries.

Worse: In the afternoon and evening, for warmth and rest.

Better: For fresh air, being outdoors, and in a cool room.

PROVEN INDICATORS FOR CEPA

Colds, whooping cough in the early stages, conjunctiva and throat infections, hay fever, nerve pain after surgery and tooth extraction, and irritated bladder.

CHAMOMILLA

This is one of the most important remedies for nervous, unpleasant children and adults. Its central symptoms are extreme irritability and restlessness, overreacting, and a low tolerance for pain.

CHARACTERISTIC SYMPTOMS

Mental/Emotional: Restless and impatient. Pitiful, stubborn, flippant, and angry. Very moody; nothing is right; children want to be carried and stroked all the time. Intolerance to pain.

Head: Pounding headache; head is hot; damp/cold sweat on the forehead and scalp. One cheek is red, the other pale and cold. Facial muscles twitch, including those of the lips and tongue. Stabbing pain in the jaw and teeth, radiating into the ears, W: for warm drinks, coffee, at night, and for being pregnant. B: for drinking ice-cold water. Toothache, W: in a warm room, B: for movement and cold drinks.

Sensory Organs: Extreme, stabbing earaches and ear ringing. Ear is swollen, as if clogged; it is sore, hot, and drives the patient crazy. Nose is irritated, clogged up, and there are constant sneezing attacks; very sensitive to smells.

Breathing Organs: Throat is irritated, as if "squeezed together" with a feeling as if a lump is stuck in the throat; throat glands are swollen. Larynx scratchy; hoarse, forced to clear throat with a feeling of tightness in the chest. Mucus rattles in children, heavy mucus formation with a bitter taste, difficult to cough up.

Digestion: Stabbing pain in the pit of the stomach; frequent, foul-tasting burping. Digestive problems after unpleasantness. Too much coffee causes nausea. Sweating attacks when drinking and eating. Stabbing pain from flatulence up into the chest. Pulling, pinching pain from the navel into the back. Flatulence with colic, hot perspiration, and red cheeks. Hot diarrhea after angry outbreaks with extreme, foul-smelling gas; the diarrhea has a greenish consistency, like spinach. Diarrhea during teething. Rectum is sore; painful hemorrhoids.

Menstruation: Heavy, with dark-colored blood; contraction-like, unbearable pain.

Sleep: Nightmares with half-opened eyes; cries and whimpering during sleep.

Worse: At night, for heat, anger, being outdoors, in the wind, and for coffee.

Better: For humid warmth (compresses, weather); for children—being carried around and driving in a car.

PROVEN INDICATORS FOR CHAMOMILLA

Irritability, nervous restlessness, nervous headaches, migraines, facial neuralgia, sleep disturbances, earaches and toothaches, difficulty during teething, diaper rash, nervous stomach, intestinal problems, hemorrhoids, and menstrual cramps.

CHINA

China has proven effective treating exhaustion, particularly after loss of fluids and severe illnesses. An important symptom is the periodic return of the problem.

CHARACTERISTIC SYMPTOMS

Mental/Emotional: Irritable, depressed, and indifferent. Sudden angry screaming, followed by being friendly and happy. Easily discouraged, lack of concentration, mental work is difficult. Can't stand loud noise.

Head: Heavy, pounding or bursting headache from temple to temple, W: for being outdoors, in bright light, for smells, and noise. B: for pressure, especially a tight compress around the head. Scalp is extremely sensitive. Face is swollen and yellowish or red. Everything tastes salty.

Sensory Organs: Has hearing difficulty. Has noise in ears. Vision problems with pressure on the eyes. Has nosebleeds, severe sneezing attacks, and is very sensitive to smells.

Breathing Organs: Mucus rattles. Severe attacks of a hacking cough after laughing and eating. Has difficulty breathing, *W:* in the evening.

Digestion: Burps frequently, which taste bitter and bring no relief. Heartburn. Lacks appetite but is ravenously hungry. Desires sweet and sour tastes, coffee and alcohol, but can't handle either. Constant flatulence with visibly distended abdomen; has breathing difficulty and heart palpitation, particularly after fruit. Rumbling in the abdomen with severe gas. Digestion is slow, and stool contains undigested food. Stabbing pain in the rectum.

Menstruation: Too early and too heavy, in large clumps. Lower abdomen is visibly distended, painful; possibly has fainting attacks. Has discharge in the middle of the cycle, which contains strings of blood.

Male Genitalia: Energy-robbing semen discharge.

Extremities/Back: Limbs and joints are painful as if sprained, can't tolerate touch. Area of the lower back is painful when lying down. Cutting pain throughout the spine, radiating into the head.

Skin: Extremely sensitive to touch, *B:* pressure.

Fever: Varied, returns periodically with shivers. Heavy perspiration at the slightest exertion. Night sweats.

Worse: During the night, in the morning, for gentle touch, for draft, loss of body fluids, after eating, bending down, and every other day.

Better: For strong pressure, stretching, being outdoors, and for warmth.

PROVEN INDICATORS FOR CHINA

Headaches due to overwork and exhaustion, heartburn, feeling bloated, flatulence, and menstrual problems.

CIMICIFUGA

One of the main remedies for muscle pain and cramps of the uterus, *Cimicifuga* is often helpful before and during menstruation. It is also given as preparation for birth as well as for pain relief during and after birth. It is suggested that this remedy be taken during pregnancy and at birth only after consultation with your physician and midwife.

CHARACTERISTIC SYMPTOMS

Mental/Emotional: Distinct physical and mental/emotional restlessness, very talkative, changes the subject all the time. Mood swings; sad, sorrowful, fears disaster, then again joyful and playful. *W:* before menstruation. *B:* at the onset of menstruation.

Head: Pain starts in the back of the head, often on the left side, pushing to the outside; also migraine-like. Feeling as if the brain is opening up and closing again; frequently helpful during menstruation and menopause.

Sensory Organs: Eyes are painful, as if "pressed together." Cannot tolerate artificial light. Ears are ringing; very sensitive to noise.

Heart: Heart palpitations with pain that radiates into the left arm.

Digestion: Nausea and vomiting, particularly during menstruation.

Uterus: Before and during menstruation, painful cramps vertically through the pelvis from one hip to the other and up into the chest. Pain in the ovaries, radiating into the abdomen and thighs. Strong after-contraction, can't handle the pain anymore.

Menstruation: Too early, too late, heavy or sparse; the pain increases with increased bleeding.

Extremities: Shooting or cramp-like muscle and joint pain, stiff.

Worse: In the morning, for cold (except headaches).

Better: For warmth and eating.

PROVEN INDICATORS FOR CIMICIFUGA

Premenstrual complaints with headaches or migraines, painful, heavy, or irregular menstruation, preparation for birth, regulating contraction activities, relieving pain during and after birth.

COCCULUS

Cocculus is an important remedy for the treatment of primarily nerve-related complaints, symptoms that generally appear along with a lack of motivation and feelings of numbness. Complaints get worse when eating and drinking.

CHARACTERISTIC SYMPTOMS

Mental/Emotional: Sad, talks little, is easily offended, absent-minded, shy, and gentle. Particularly well suited after worry and grief. Easily overburdened and slow to understand. Time passes too quickly.

Head: Pain in the back of the head and forehead with nausea and constant dizziness due to worry, lack of sleep, overwork, and driving. Facial neuralgia, W: in the afternoon. The complexion is greenish-yellow.

Digestion: Motion sickness. An aversion to food and the smell of food and tobacco smoke. A painful, visibly distended abdomen causes awakening at midnight. Colic from flatulence, particularly during pregnancy, B: lying down on alternate sides.

Menstruation: Irregular, too early, substantial, dark, lumpy, with painful pressure on the uterus, and cutting, contracting pain; severe, overall weakness during menstruation, can hardly remain upright.

Extremities/Back: Hands shake while eating, and the higher the hand is moved, the worse it gets. Hands and arms fall asleep easily. Weak, cracking knees. Back feels paralyzed, and shoulders and arms feel as if they are bruised.

Sleep: Yawning cramps. Insomnia in spite of being overly tired; particularly for people who work at night and nursing mothers.

Worse: In the afternoon, for eating, lack of sleep, noises, loud noises, menstruation, and emotional stress.

Better: For lying down and quiet.

PROVEN INDICATORS FOR COCCULUS
Headaches after overwork, sadness, depression, tiredness, fatigue, exhaustion, insomnia, nervous stomach, intestinal problems, morning sickness and vomiting during pregnancy, irregular painful menstruation, and motion sickness.

COFFEA

Coffea is a remedy that specifically addresses the central nervous system. Its central symptoms are great excitability and a low tolerance for pain. These symptoms can be caused by too much coffee. The best remedy is to reduce consumption!

CHARACTERISTIC SYMPTOMS
Mental/Emotional: Mentally overstimulated, one thought is chasing the next. Intelligent, a quick learner, but has little patience. Easily excited, can't sleep, even joyful events overexcite. Happy. Laughs and cries at the same time. Always on the move. Can't tolerate even the slightest pain.

Head: Stabbing headaches, as if from a nail. Also facial neuralgia due to exposure to cold wind, W: outdoors.

Face: Dry and hot, with red cheeks.

Sensory Organs: Overly sensitive to smells and sounds. Can hear the faintest, but also nonexisting, sounds.

Mouth: Unbearable toothaches, B: for drinking ice-cold water and sucking on ice.

Heart: Irregular heartbeat, particularly after happy surprises.

Digestion: Very hungry, can't stand anything tight around the waist.

Female Genitalia: Strong vaginal itching, elevated libido.

Menstruation: Too early, too long, light red or dark, with clumps.

Sleep: "Thinking" too much interferes with falling asleep. Wakes up early in the morning and is then only able to doze. *W:* wine.

Worse: At night, for cold air, cold wind; excitement, smells, noise; for being outdoors, for motion, wine, and coffee.

Better: For warmth, lying down, and sucking on ice.

PROVEN INDICATORS FOR COFFEA

Nervous restlessness, being overly active; sleep disturbances, headaches, neuralgia, toothaches, and menstrual problems.

COLOCYNTHIS

The central symptom of *Colocynthis* is severe neuralgic pain, primarily in the head and abdomen, that can most always be lessened by applying pressure. It is especially suitable for people who are easily irritated, angry, and have a tendency to be overweight.

CHARACTERISTIC SYMPTOMS

Mental/Emotional: Very irritated. Can't handle being questioned. Angry, even outraged when being questioned or if feels an insult.

Head: Severe, pounding or burning pain in the right temple or the left half of the head, *B:* warmth. Dizzy from moving the head suddenly. Facial neuralgia, particularly on the left side, *B:* strong pressure.

Sensory Organs: Cutting pain in the eye, *W:* bending down. Eyelid twitches. Hears an echo sound in the ears.

Teeth: Feels as if teeth are too long. Stomach pain always appears with headache and a toothache.

Digestion: Bitter taste in the mouth, and cutting, agonizing pain in the abdomen, forcing the person to bend over, *W:* for eating fruit or walking. *B:* for pressure. Thin, jelly-like, yellow stool after unpleasant events, fruit and ice-cold drinks, and when the body is overheated.

Urinary Tract: Frequent urge to urinate, but urine is sparse. Burning sensation in the whole abdomen when urinating. Kidney pain, particularly on the left side.

Menstruation: Delayed, repressed periods with cramp-like pain, *B:* from drastically bending over. Cramps in the left ovary and uterus.

Extremities/Back: Cramps from the hips to the knees, particularly on the left side, B: from sitting or from lying down on the painful side. Muscles feel as if they are "wrapped up tight." Sudden, severe pain attacks in the pelvis, back, and hips, B: from bending over.

Worse: In the evening, at night, for excitement, eating, and drinking.

Better: Bending over, applying strong pressure, rest, lying on the painful side, warmth.

PROVEN INDICATORS FOR COLOCYNTHIS

Irritability, headaches, facial neuralgia, diarrhea, nervous stomach, intestinal problems, cystitis, kidney colic, and menstrual cramps.

DULCAMARA

This remedy is indispensable for complaints that appear during damp/cold late-summer weather and for colds that produce a severe mucus discharge. It also can be helpful in cases of rheumatic pain.

CHARACTERISTIC SYMPTOMS

Mental/Emotional: Confusion.

Head: Back of the head is painful, heavy, and cool because of exposure to cold. There are brown scales on the scalp that bleed when scratched. Facial neuralgia due to exposure to cold.

Sensory Organs: Cold affects eyes, W: outdoors. Pain in the ears. Nose is clogged due to exposure to cold/rain. Tongue is rough and scratchy. Lips are sore.

Breathing Organs: Dry or mucus-producing cough. Also a cramp-like cough and a whooping cough that produces a lot of mucus. Has a torturous, dry cough in the winter. Coughs after physical exertion.

Digestion: An aversion to food, but an extreme, burning desire for cold water. Stabbing pain in the area of the navel. Heartburn, nausea, and vomiting with shivers. Yellow-greenish diarrhea when the weather is damp and cold.

Urinary Tract: Frequent urge to urinate after sitting on a cold surface (sitting on a cold seat, cold rocks, or a cold floor).

Extremities/Back: Feet are ice-cold and hands are sweaty. Neck and shoulder area is heavy, lame, and stiff when weather is damp and cold. A lame back.

Skin: Dry. Urticaria rash due to cold or sour food. Eczema before menstruation. Constant itching in damp/cold weather.

Worse: Damp/cold of any kind.

Better: Warmth (external) and movement.

PROVEN INDICATORS FOR DULCAMARA
Sensitivity to weather changes, colds, facial neuralgia, ear pain, rash, stomach and intestinal problems, cystitis, and a whooping cough.

EUPHRASIA

Euphrasia is the most important remedy for eye problems. Its central symptoms are biting tears but a mild cold.

CHARACTERISTIC SYMPTOMS
Head: Dull headaches from a cold with a heavy flow of tears and mucus discharge from the nose. Severe, bursting headaches in which the eyes feel as if "blinded." Face is hot and red. Upper lip feels stiff.
Eyes: Conjunctiva irritation due to draft, conjunctivitis. Eyes are "swimming" in watery, acid-like tears. Thick, sore-producing discharge from eyes. Sticky mucus clogs eyelids, interfering with vision. Blinks eyes constantly.
Nose: Profuse, thin, watery discharge.
Breathing Organs: Severe cough with heavy mucus expelled, sometimes with vomiting. A whooping cough with heavy tear flow, during day only.
Skin: Early stages of measles in which the eyes are affected.
Worse: For sunlight, bright artificial light, warm winds, and warm rooms.
Better: For rubbing, darkness, and coffee.

PROVEN INDICATORS FOR EUPHRASIA
Colds, hay fever, stressed eyes, conjunctivitis, early stages of measles, and whooping cough.

FERRUM PHOSPHORICUM

Ferrum phosphoricum is an important remedy for the early stages of colds and illnesses involving fever. Complaints increase swiftly but not as suddenly as with *Aconitum* and *Belladonna*. Central symptoms are distinct weakness and an anemic complexion alternating with temporary flushing and an urge toward movement.

CHARACTERISTIC SYMPTOMS
Mental/Emotional: Nervous, irritated, and sensitive. Can't tolerate noise.
Head: Severe, pounding headache, often with dizziness, often after expo-

sure to too much sun, B: nosebleed. Very sensitive to touch, B: for cold compresses. Face is red, and cheeks are hot and sore. Facial neuralgia, W: for bending down or shaking the head.

Sensory Organs: Eyes are red and burn painfully. Hearing is difficult; there are ear noises; the outer part of the ear is red. Nosebleeds light red, particularly in the early stages of a cold.

Breathing Organs: Throat is red and sore, ulcerated. Tonsils are red and swollen. Sore throat due to too much singing and talking. Has a short, croup-like, painful, cramp-like cough, that also tickles, W: outdoors and at night. Feels a stabbing pain when breathing deep into the chest. Has a whooping cough with hoarseness or a total loss of voice.

Digestion: A changing appetite. Sour burping, heartburn, and an aversion to milk and meat. Stomach pain after eating, due to pressure. Vomiting of undigested food with gallbladder fluids. Has urges for stimulants. Watery stool containing undigested food. Hemorrhoids.

Urinary Tract: Incontinence when coughing.

Extremities/Back: Stiff neck and rheumatic pain in the shoulder radiating into chest and hands. Palms are hot, and hands painfully swollen. Back is tense.

Skin: Night sweats in cases of anemia.

Sleep: Restless, has nightmares.

Worse: In the evening, nights, early in the morning, and motion.*

Better: Lying down, using cold, and motion.*

PROVEN INDICATORS FOR FERRUM PHOSPHORICUM
Colds, flus, earaches, nosebleeds, and whooping cough.

GELSEMIUM

Gelsemium is the main remedy for colds and illnesses with a fever, and it is also suitable for nervous complaints that develop slowly. Its central symptoms are distinct tiredness and an anxious weakness with tremors and dizziness.

CHARACTERISTIC SYMPTOMS
Mental/Emotional: Numb, indifferent. Anxiously excited or without any fear at all. Stage fright. Weak memory and concentration. Wants to be left alone.

*Motion can worsen *or* improve the symptoms.

207

Head: Pressure headaches, like a belt fastened tightly around the head. Pain radiates into ears and chin with vision problems and dizziness. Also, pain in the back of the head, radiating into neck and shoulders. *B:* pressure and elevating the head. If there is fever, the face is red, hot, and heavy.

Sensory Organs: Eyes are bloodshot, with vision problems. Pain above and inside the eyes. Weak eye muscles with dizziness and double vision; heavy eyelids. Ear pain that originates in the throat, hearing problems. Cold with runny nose, tickling, and a feeling of "fullness" at the base of the nose. Tongue is numb and jittery; the person can't talk properly.

Breathing Organs: Bad breath. The sense of having a lump in the throat; difficulty swallowing. Throat and tonsils are sore and swollen. Pain from the throat to the ears. Dry cough with a runny nose. Slow breathing with a sense of weakness and a feeling of apprehension in the chest. Loss of voice.

Heart: A sense as if the heart is going to stop beating unless one is in constant motion.

Digestion: Absence of thirst and an empty feeling in the pit of the stomach. Nervous diarrhea due to excitement or fear. Stool and urine incontinence.

Menstruation: Too late, too sparse, pain radiates into the back and hips.

Extremities/Back: Painful limbs and muscle weakness. Jittery hands and feet. A deep-seated, dull backache, as if bruised. Every exertion is too much.

Skin: Hot and dry. Measle-like rash with itching.

Sleep: Restless, anxious. Sleepless due to exhaustion.

Fever: Extreme jitters, wants to be held.

Worse: In the A.M., for humid weather, fog, before a thunderstorm, during a change of weather, for excitement, emotional stress, and nicotine.

Better: For fresh air, motion, frequent urination, sitting up, sitting back, and stimulants.

PROVEN INDICATORS FOR GELSEMIUM
Stage fright, test anxiety, motion sickness, sleep disturbances, colds, flus, headaches, migraine headaches, muscle and joint pain, and measles.

HAMAMELIS

Hamamelis is an indispensable remedy for venous hematomas, particularly hemorrhoids and varicose veins. All complaints are aggregated when exposed to warmth, humid air, motion, and during menstruation. It is also useful in the form of salve or tincture for external application.

HEPAR SULFURIS

One of the main remedies for a festering process. Its central symptoms are a great need for warmth and a strong tendency to catch cold; all symptoms get worse when exposed to cold.

CHARACTERISTIC SYMPTOMS

Mental/Emotional: Overly sensitive, easily angered, has tamper tantrums, and is quarrelsome. Needs constant diversion but is always dissatisfied. Talks fast and is in a hurry. Even minimal pain is considered unbearable.

Head: Facial neuralgia on the right side. Upper lip is cracked.

Sensory Organs: Eyes are red, inflamed, thick, festering; a yellow discharge clogs the eyelids in the morning; very sensitive to light. Pointed, stabbing pain in the ears and has a hearing disturbance when blowing nose; festering discharge. Outer ear is red, hot, and itches. Runny nose with sneezing attacks after exposure to cold wind, and there is an ample, green/yellowish mucus discharge from the nose. Sense of smell is either exaggerated or lost. Unpleasant, foul-smelling mouth odor, ample saliva; festering ulcers in the mouth cavity, bitter taste in the mouth.

Breathing Organs: Pain in the throat as if from a splinter that radiates pain into the ears. Problems swallowing. Dangerous infection of the tonsils. Three types of cough: dry, hoarse, W: walking. Dry and rattling, W: cold, draft. Croaking, suffocating cough in which the person bends the head down to be able to get air, W: dry, cold air.

Digestion: Loves sour and piquant foods and has aversion against fat. Nausea in the morning with frequent burping that produces no taste or smell. Heavy feeling in the stomach even after a light meal. Stool is sour, foul-smelling, and undigested. Even soft stool is difficult to pass.

Skin: Does not heal well, every small injury festering. Broken skin, particularly on hands and feet. Bad complexion with festering pimples. Heavy perspiration, sticky, foul-smelling, sour, particularly with a fever.

Worse: Toward morning, for cold, draft, and touch. Worse for lying down on the painful side.

Better: For warmth, being wrapped up, and in damp weather.

PROVEN INDICATORS FOR HEPAR SULFURIS

Sensitivity to changes in the weather, sinus infections, throat problems, laryngitis, abscesses, and boils.

HYPERICUM

Next to *Arnica*, *Hypericum* is the most important remedy for injuries of nerve-rich tissue, like bruises and contusions on the nails and fingers, complaints after dental treatment, and following surgery and giving birth. It is also available in the form of a tincture for external use.

IGNATIA

Ignatia is very effective for treating the aftermath of worries and sorrow, also lovesickness. Its central symptoms are extreme sensitivity of the sensory organs and intolerance to tobacco smoke.

CHARACTERISTIC SYMPTOMS
Mental/Emotional: Quick mood changes. Introverted, withdrawn, silent, depressed, melancholy, and whiny. Sighs and cries a lot. Sleeplessness due to sorrow.

Head: Nervous headache as if stuck by a nail. Tension headaches after unpleasant events, fighting, grief, or during menstruation; frequently associated with vision problems. Muscle twitches in the face. Facial color changes during rest.

Sensory Organs: Sour taste in the mouth, W: coffee, smoking. Quick to bite the inside of the cheek.

Breathing Organs: Stabbing pain or a lump in the throat, B: solid food. A dry, cramp-like cough with much sighing.

Digestion: Sour burping, heavy flatulence, a feeling of fullness, burping, and hiccups. A stabbing, colic-like abdominal pain, often one-sided. Stabbing pain in the rectum, from the inside out or with a sense of tightness after passing stool. Hemorrhoids, anal prolapse. Diarrhea or constipation due to emotional stress, or due to an appetite for rich, fatty foods.

Urinary Tract: Substantial, watery urine; holds back urination during menstruation.

Menstruation: Too early, too weak, or too heavy, and dark to black in color; has menstrual cramps, and feels very exhausted and tired.

Extremities: Limbs twitch and has lower leg cramps, particularly during sleep.

Skin: Very sensitive to cold drafts, has tendency to have allergic rashes and itching.

Worse: In the morning, outdoors, after eating, for coffee, nicotine, tobacco smoke, excitement, and external warmth.
Better: While eating, changing position.

PROVEN INDICATORS FOR IGNATIA

Sadness, depression, mood changes, sleep disturbances, nervous headaches, catarrh headaches, stomach and intestinal problems, menstrual problems, nausea during pregnancy, and problems with nursing. IMPORTANT: *Ignatia* does not go together with *Coffea, Nux vomica,* or *Tabacum;* do not use these remedies in succession!

KALI BICHROMICUM

This remedy is used to treat colds with a discharge of thick, gummy mucus from the soft tissues. It has also been effective for rheumatic complaints and is especially suited for phlegmatic children and adults.

CHARACTERISTIC SYMPTOMS

Mental/Emotional: Tired, exhausted.
Head: Headaches with nausea, dizziness when getting up, often preceded by vision problems. Stabbing pain that moves about, particularly in the forehead. Sensitive scalp.
Sensory Organs: Eyelids are swollen and inflamed, gummed up with yellow, stringy discharge. Heavy tearing, very sensitive to light. Stabbing ear pain, particularly on the left side. Children have a constantly runny nose. A cold with thick, sticky, greenish-yellow mucus, forming strings; the mucus sticks in the throat. Also for chronic sinus infections with a stuffed nose. Ulcers on the soft tissue in the nose, holes in the septum, as if punched out. Tongue with yellow coating or bright red, dry, ridges like a road map.
Breathing Organs: Throat is tight, red, inflamed, and the tonsils and lymph nodes behind ears are swollen. Rattling cough moves thick, stringy slime.
Digestion: Stomach has griping pains, and there is flatulence directly after eating. Slimy vomiting. Loves beer, but can't tolerate it.
Urinary Tract: Feeling as if the last drop of urine is held back.
Extremities/Back: Stomach problems alternate with rheumatic complaints. Rheumatic pains come and go quickly, move throughout the body, often only in small areas and joints. Pain radiates far into the back and coccyx.
Worse: In the morning; for cold air, damp weather (cold); hot weather, and changes in the weather (rheumatic pain).

Better: For warmth and movement (rheumatic pain but not sciatic pain).

PROVEN INDICATORS FOR KALI BICHROMICUM
Colds, sinus infections, stomach and intestinal upset, rheumatic complaints, and sensitivity to changes in the weather.

LACHESIS

Lachesis is a far-reaching remedy with emphasis on mental/emotional issues and is appropriate for both men and women. Its central symptoms are that the person can't stand anything tight around the neck and body and talks all the time. Every complaint is worse after sleep. Physical problems appear primarily on the left side.

CHARACTERISTIC SYMPTOMS
Mental/Emotional: Intense mood swings. Depressed, anxious, distrustful, jealous, vengeful, and restless, *W:* in the morning. Wide awake at night and prefers to study till quite late. Talks like a "waterfall," jumping from subject to subject, can't concentrate.

Head: Neuralgic pain in the head and face, radiating into the neck and shoulder, particularly on the left side; gets dizzy when turning around and feels nauseous. Gets headaches when being in the sun too long. Facial complexion is blotchy red but also yellowish pale.

Sensory Organs: All senses are heightened and distorted. Frequent nosebleeds with a runny nose and headaches. Gums are swollen and bleed easily. Tongue is red, twitches, burns with pain, is rough with sore spots, and feels as if it has been soaped. Has a toothache that radiates into the ears.

Breathing Organs: Throat and mouth are dark red. Tonsillitis starts on the left side. Difficulty swallowing, but solid food is easier than liquid. Very sensitive to touch; can't tolerate anything tight around the neck. Suffocating cough with breathing difficulty after waking up, gasps for air, must loosen clothing and open a window.

Heart/Circulation: Awakens from the first sleep with oppressive sensations, breathing difficulty, dizziness, nausea, and anxiety or headaches.

Digestion: Gnawing hunger, must eat immediately. Preference for alcohol. Can't tolerate anything tight around the waist. Foul-smelling stool, frequent constipation with hemorrhoids, passing stool is painful.

Female Genitalia: Menstruation is irregular, too early, and sparse. premenstrual problems, *B:* when bleeding starts. Pain in the left ovary. Consider this remedy for complaints during menopause, especially hot flashes in which she perspires constantly with a strong odor. Heart races to the point of feeling as if she might faint during insomnia.

Male Genitalia: Sexually overexcited.

Extremities/Back: Pain in the coccyx, *B:* getting up. Sciatica pain, *B:* lying down. Pain in shin bone. Dark red to blackish varicose veins, open ulcers.

Skin: Hot and sweaty. The injured or inflamed area is bluish red.

Worse: In the morning, after sleeping (also when sleeping) during the day, in warm rooms, a warm bath, for hot drinks, pressure, tight clothing, in the spring, during weather and climate changes from cold to warm, for warm southern winds, humid/warm weather, and for drinking wine.

Better: For fresh air using warmth [treatment] and at the onset of menstruation.

PROVEN INDICATORS FOR LACHESIS

Sadness, depression, restlessness, insomnia, sensitivity to changes in weather, throat infections, difficulties during menstruation and menopause, insect bites, and mumps.

LEDUM

Ledum is the most important remedy for when one has been injured by needles, nails, garden tools, rakes, thorns, and insect bites. It is also good for contusions (being poked in the eye by a twig or branch) as well as for pulled ligaments and sprains. Its key symptoms are that the wound is cold, but the pain decreases from the application of cold. It is also available in tincture form for external application.

LYCOPODIUM

Lycopodium is a far-reaching remedy for mentally active but insecure and physically weakened people, as well as for children. Its central symptoms are premature aging and being a poor eater. Complaints usually begin on the right side of the body and move to the left.

CHARACTERISTIC SYMPTOMS

Mental/Emotional: Extremely irritable, can't tolerate conflict. Ambitious with a constant fear of failure. Concentration and memory problems when overworked. Children seem older than their age, precocious, and are often in a bad mood. Melancholy. Aversion to company, but afraid of loneliness. All senses are heightened.

Head: Tension headaches, particularly when not eating regularly, W: lying down. Pounding headache after coughing. Premature loss of hair; severe horizontal wrinkles on the forehead and vertical wrinkles at the base of the nose. Complexion is yellow-gray with deep circles under the eyes; turns red after eating.

Sensory Organs: Eyelids are red. Sties. Poor night vision. Sleeps with eyes halfway open. Moist eczema behind the ears; sounds in the ears reduce ability to hear. A cold with a burning, runny nose while the nose is clogged up. For sniffles in children who are awakened by them and then must rub their nose. The mouth is dry, but there is no thirst. The tongue is dry with ridges and is swollen with blisters. Toothache, B: warm drinks.

Breathing Organs: Throat and tonsils are inflamed and brown-red; the inflammation moves from the right side to the left side, W: after sleep, B: hot drinks. A hoarse cough with mucus rattling and breathing difficulties, particularly on the right side. A tickling cough during the night.

Heart: Has a feeling of apprehension when lying on the right side, particularly during the night.

Digestion: Very hungry but is full after only a few bites, often feels bloated with audible flatulence; burping and passing gas does not bring relief. Has strong urges for something sweet but does not tolerate it, becomes nervous. Can't tolerate products made from flour and starch, onions, and oysters. Everything tastes sour. Shooting pain in the stomach from right to left, can' t lie down on the right side. Constipation, hemorrhoids.

Urinary Tract: Urinating is difficult, and painful at the beginning, particularly for children. An extreme production of urine that is light, with brick-red sediment.

Male Genitalia: Premature ejaculation and difficulty with erection after intense sexual activity.

Female Genitalia: Vaginal dryness causes pain during sex. Menstrual cycle is irregular.

Back/Extremities: Burning pain between the shoulder blades; back pain when urinating. Sciatic pain on the right side. Right foot is hot, left cold. Has a heavy feeling, tingling, and numbness in the arms and legs, W: lying down, during the night. Leg cramps during the night. Chronic gout. Varicose veins.

Skin: Dry, thick, wrinkled, and spotty. Strong foot and underarm perspiration. Bad complexion and acne, W: warmth.

Worse: Right side from the top to the bottom, in the late afternoon, for warmth (also in warm bed), from hot air, and before menstruation.

Better: After midnight, for motion, hot drinks and meals, cold, and removing covers.

PROVEN INDICATORS FOR LYCOPODIUM

Irritability, fear, shyness, fatigue, exhaustion, depression, insomnia, throat infections, corns, hair loss, sluggish intestines, constipation, and flatulence.

MERCURIUS SOLUBILIS

Mercurius solubilis is one of the main remedies for festering and ulcerous wounds. All of the discharge is hot and burning; the skin is moist, and when infected, lymph nodes become swollen. For those with dry skin, *Mercurius* is not the proper remedy.

CHARACTERISTIC SYMPTOMS

Mental/Emotional: Slowed-down comprehension, answers are given reluctantly. Poor memory. Suspicious.

Head: Headaches as from a cold, as if a rope is tied around the head. Scalp feels as if stretched. A burning, foul-smelling rash on the scalp. Dizzy when lying on the back. Facial neuralgia due to cold wind, pulling pain.

Sensory Organs: Eyelids are sore and red; thick, sharp, burning, festering discharge makes eyelids stick together. Very sensitive to light. Stabbing pain in the ears. A cold with a runny nose and frequent sneezing. Thick, yellowish-green, sharp, burning discharge from the nose. Nose is sore. Sneezing attacks when exposed to light.

Mouth: Toothache, W: during the night. Teeth are loose, decayed. Gums are swollen, bleed at the slightest touch; neck of tooth is exposed; festering sores and ulcers in the mouth cavity and tongue; burning, stabbing pain. Tongue is limp, twitching, moist, and thick with yellow coating, has deep vertical ridges and indentations from the teeth. A great deal of saliva. Bad breath.

Breathing Organs: Throat and tonsils are red, also ulcerated, with burning, stabbing pain. Must swallow constantly. Severe coughing attacks during the night; coughs up thick, yellow-green mucus, W: lying on the right side, tobacco smoke. Has also a whooping cough and nosebleeds.

Digestion: Strong thirst for cold drinks. Aversion to bread, butter, wine, and strong alcohol. Constantly hungry but has poor digestion, flatulence, burping, feels full, stomach pain; frequently passes stool, but produces only small amounts, and has a feeling of never being finished.

Urinary Tract: Frequent urges to urinate but produces only a few drops. Burning pain in the urethra during urination.

Extremities: Hands are weak and shake on exerting effort. Joints are weak.

Skin: Always almost damp. Perspires easily and profusely. Itches, *W:* in a warm bed.

Worse: During the night, in humid/wet weather, for draft, warm rooms, and in a warm bed.

Better: Moderate temperatures.

PROVEN INDICATORS FOR MERCURIUS SOLUBILIS

Poor memory and concentration, throat infections, cystitis, whooping cough, and difficulty with nursing. IMPORTANT: *Mercurius solubilis* does not go well with many otherhomeopathic remedies; for that reason, use it only after consultation with and the approval of your homeopath.

NATRUM CHLORATUM

Natrum chloratum is a very valuable remedy for the treatment of many of the after-effects of deep-seated worry and pain, as well as anemia. Its central symptoms are distinct weakness in the morning before getting out of bed and between 10 and 11 A.M., a great tendency toward catching colds, constantly being cold, and an aversion toward medication.

CHARACTERISTIC SYMPTOMS

Mental/Emotional: introverted, sad, serious, loyal, sacrifices for others but is not holding grudges; moody. Tends to overdramatize. Sheds tears when laughing. Buries self in old hurt and pain, can't tolerate sympathy, wants to be left alone but then cries. Can't sleep because of worry. Depressed, anxious, afraid to make a fool of self. Heart races with fear in small rooms and in crowds; has a tendency to faint.

Head: Bursting, burning headaches from sunup to sundown, particularly young girls and in the presence of anemia after menstruation. Also chronic headaches and migraines with dizziness and nausea. The lips, nose, and lower jaw are numb, tingling. Complexion is pale, oily, and shiny.

Sensory Organs: Eyelids heavy, feel as if "bruised," letters blur into each other. Sharp, burning tears. Coughing causes eyes to water. A cold with a watery, runny nose and severe sneezing at the beginning of the cold; later the nose gets clogged up, and it secretes a substance that is like raw egg white. Nose is sore inside. Sinus infection. Pearl-like blisters on the lips; lips and the corners of the mouth are dry, cracked, with deep cracks in the lower lip. Tongue is coated with foam and has ridges "like those on a topical map."

Breathing Organs: Short of breath when exerting effort and climbing stairs.

Digestion: Extremely thirsty, has great urges for salt, something salty, and perspires when eating. Has an aversion to sour foods, bread, fat, slimy food, and aspic. Hard, dry, lumpy stool causes bleeding from the rectum.

Female Genitalia: Itches; vagina is dry and sex painful.

Menstruation: Irregular and too heavy.

Urinary Tract: Cannot urinate in the presence of others.

Extremities/Back: Severe pain in the lower back. Legs are weak, cold, and make noise when moving. Numbness and tingling in arms and legs. Skin of palms is greasy, oily. Has crust buildup at the hairline, behind the ears, inside the elbows, and behind the knees. Has warts on the palms. Dermatitis, *B*: salt, at the seashore.

Worse: In the morning, in warm rooms, for heat, noise, music, lying down, given sympathy (but B also possible!), and mental stress.

Better: For being outdoors, a cold bath, tight clothes, and lying on the right side.

PROVEN INDICATORS FOR NATRUM CHLORATUM
Sadness, depression, fear, sleeping problems, migraines, a bad complexion, nettle fever, sun allergies, colds that start with severe sneezing attacks, sinus infections, stomach and intestinal problems, and problems with menopause.

NUX VOMICA

Today, *Nux vomica* is the most used remedy; it addresses all the complaints indicative of our hectic, performance-oriented society. It is particularly well suited to people whose activities are primarily mental and are performed in a sitting position. It is also useful after the misuse of medications and stimulants (nicotine, coffee, and alcohol).

CHARACTERISTIC SYMPTOMS
Mental/Emotional: Impatient, bad tempered, competitive, pedantic, and hypochrondriacal. Easily frightened, has anxiety attacks. Tendency to mis-

use medication and stimulants. A very low tolerance to pain. Is highly sensitive to cold.

Head: Headaches in the forehead, B: pressure. Neck pain with dizziness. Roaring pain in the head. Dizziness with brief losses of consciousness, W: in the morning and late in the evening. Has headaches after too much food, alcohol, or sun.

Sensory Organs: Highly sensitive to light, noises, and smells. Itches inside the ears. Has a runny nose in the morning, but it is clogged up at night. Has nosebleeds in the morning. A remedy good for sniffling in young children after exposure to dry cold. Tongue is covered with a white coating. Has a bad taste in the mouth.

Breathing Organs: Hoarseness; has a rough, scratchy throat. Throat tickles upon waking up in the morning. Coughing causes bursting headaches. Shallow breathing with feeling of apprehension.

Digestion: Nauseated in the morning, particularly after a late meal the night before. Food sits in the stomach like a stone, has a feeling of fullness; burping has a sour, bitter taste; heartburn, flatulence, and nausea; vomiting urges are unsuccessful 1 to 2 hours after eating, W: coffee. Loves fatty foods and can handle them. Abdomen is very sensitive to pressure, must loosen clothing. Diarrhea after too much food, otherwise has a tendency toward constipation with frequent but unsuccessful attempts to pass stool. Painful, bloody hemorrhoids.

Urinary Tract: Irritated bladder.

Menstruation: Irregular, too early, too long, dark to blackish, often fainting attacks, backaches, and constipation.

Male Genitalia: Easily excitable libido.

Extremities/Back: Lumbago, almost impossible to turn in bed. Sudden weakness in the arms and legs; falls asleep easily. Knee creaks when moving. Cramps in lower legs and soles of the feet.

Skin: Red, spotty, with frequent occurrences of acne. Burning, hot rash with digestive problems; difficulty moving, shivers when losing bed covers.

Sleep: Awakens around 3 A.M. and remains awake until the early-morning hours. Feels terrible when waking up. Has dreams of work and time pressures.

Worse: In the morning, for job- and money-related worries, for light, noises, smells, cold, draft, being outdoors, dry weather, touch, after eating, alcohol, nicotine, coffee, and tranquilizers.

Better: In the evening, short naps, rest/quiet, damp warmth, and pressure.

PROVEN INDICATORS FOR NUX VOMICA

Irritability, fear, panic attacks, sleeping problems, nervous headaches, headaches due to overworking and muscle tension, problems resulting from a hangover, sensitivity to changes in the weather, colds, hay fever, throat infections, toothaches, sensitive teeth, stomach and intestinal problems, and cystitis. IMPORTANT: *Nux vomica* does not get along with *Coffea*, *Ignatia*, *Cocculus*, and *Zincum metallicum*; do not take these remedies in succession!

PHOSPHORUS

Phosphorus is an indispensable remedy for the effects of nervous overload, particularly when the senses are flooded with stimuli; also where there is a tendency to bleed. It is especially appropriate for tall, slender people with transparent skin.

CHARACTERISTIC SYMPTOMS

Mental/Emotional: A very fine antenna for external stimuli; everything is felt keenly; wants to do everything at once. Little perseverance, restless, and fragile. Intelligent, imaginative, helpful, and communicative. For cases of overstimulation, stubbornness, melancholy, apathy. Loves company. Has great fear of being alone, thunderstorms, illness, darkness, and bad luck.

Head: Dizzy when getting up, especially older people. Tension headaches with a cold feeling in the neck, but hot along the spine. Feels as if the brain "is tired." Hair falls out in bunches, bare spots on the scalp; dandruff with itching. A pale complexion, transparent with bluish circles under the eyes.

Sensory Organs: All senses are highly charged. Visual problems with a diminished field of vision when reading and blurred long-distance vision. Auditory problems, particularly relating to human voices; hears echoes. Nose is dry and painfully swollen. For chronic colds with bloody, yellow-greenish slimy discharge, and ulcers inside the nose. Nose polyps. Nosebleeds. Tongue is chalk-white with a red stripe in the middle.

Mouth: Frequently bleeding gums, particularly when brushing teeth. Gums are ulcerated and receding.

Breathing Organs: Hoarseness; throat is sore, scratchy, very painful; the person can hardly talk; burning scratching pain when swallowing. Palate and tonsils are dark red. A severe dry cough with burning chest pain and a sweet-tasting discharge. Tightness in the chest, feeling as if something is sitting on top of the chest.

Digestion: Nervous stomach, especially when eating unfamiliar food and during climate changes; sour-tasting burping after eating, sometimes also burping up undigested food; stomachaches, nausea, vomiting, W: warm food and drinks; can handle only cold water, cold food, and ice. Painless diarrhea after excitement, followed by feeling very weak. Stool and gas are very foul-smelling.

Extremities/Back: Jittery, weak arms and legs after exertion. Burning pain between the shoulder blades.

Skin: Itching, burning rash after eating fish. Allergic reaction to penicillin. A tendency to bruise easily. Even small injuries bleed heavily and break open again.

Worse: In the evening, during the night, for light, noise, twilight, smells, touch, thunderstorms, changes in the weather or climate, warm food and drinks, and stress of any kind.

Better: For darkness, being outdoors, cold food and drinks, cold, rest/quiet, and sleep.

PROVEN INDICATORS FOR PHOSPHORUS

Fear, phobias, overactivity, memory and concentration problems, insomnia, nervous headaches, fatigue, exhaustion, tiredness, laryngitis, nervous stomach and intestinal problems, allergic dermatitis, and hair loss. IMPORTANT: *Phosphorus* does not combine well with *Causticum*; do not take these remedies in succession!.

PHYTOLACCA

Phytolacca is a valuable remedy for treating infected glands and rheumatic complaints. Its central symptoms are hard, swollen glands and a sensitivity to changes in the weather. Complaints usually start on the right side.

CHARACTERISTIC SYMPTOMS

Head: Pressure headaches in the forehead and temples, radiating into the back of the head. Dizziness when getting up, sensitive scalp. W: weather changes, particularly when changing to damp/cold.

Sensory Organs: Eyes are painful: feels as if there is sand under the eyelids. There is an abundant production of hot tears. A cold with slimy discharge from only one side of the nose; postnasal drip.

Breathing Organs: The palate, throat, and tonsils are dark red to bluish and swollen. The throat is scratchy, dry, tight, and hot; burning pain when swallowing, which radiates into the ears. Ear/saliva glands are enlarged and sensitive to touch or as hard as stones and swollen (as in mumps).

Female Breasts: The breasts are sore, rough, and inflamed, swollen, hard as stones, and very painful; the pain when nursing radiates throughout the body.

Extremities/Back: The neck and back are stiff when waking up in the morning, W: damp weather. Pain shoots from the lower back into the soles of the feet. Rheumatic, burning pain shoots throughout the whole body like electrical shock waves, W: during the night, during a storm. Severe pain in the heels, B: elevating feet above the head.

Worse: During the night, damp/cold weather, and changes in the weather.

Better: For warm, dry weather, and rest/quiet.

PROVEN INDICATORS FOR PHYTOLACCA

Sensitivity to changes in the weather, throat infections, tonsillitis, mumps, and breast inflammation (mastitis) during nursing. IMPORTANT: *Phytolacca* does not work with *Mercurius solubilis*; do not take these remedies in succession.

PULSATILLA

Pulsatilla is a remedy that has far-reaching effects and is particularly effective for clinging children and gentle, sensitive people who are guided by their feelings and need of a lot of attention. Its central symptoms are moodiness and complaints that change constantly and are often contradictory. For example, the person gets chilled easily but can't stand warmth in any form. Complaints often start on the right side and improve when given fresh air, attention, and sympathy.

CHARACTERISTIC SYMPTOMS

Mental/Emotional: The mood changes like the weather in April. Very sensitive, good-hearted, helpful, gentle, shy, sentimental, and romantic, but also dependent, fearful, indecisive, and whiny. Needs lot of attention, acknowledgment, and sympathy, otherwise will become moody, dissatisfied, complain, be distrustful, jealous, easily offended, insolent, stubborn, and smug. Fears being left alone, darkness, ghosts, and the future. Has anxiety attacks with a tendency to faint when in a crowd or in close spaces. During a crisis, usually strong and resolute.

Head: "Wandering" pain in the forehead and above the eyes; head feels as if bursting apart, often on the right side, with dizziness. Facial neuralgia on the right side with eye tearing.

Sensory Organs: Itching and burning eyes. Eyelids are inflamed with a lot of thick, yellow, mild, slimy discharge. Sties. Exposed parts of the ears are swollen and red. Pain in the beginning is light. Does not hear well; feels as if the ears are clogged up. Has a mild cold with a thick, yellow or yellow-greenish discharge. Often starts on the right side. Moving between indoors and outdoors causes frequent changes from a runny nose to a clogged-up nose. The tongue's coating is yellow or white and slimy. Taste in the mouth changes constantly between bitter, salty, and foul.

Mouth: Dry but not thirsty.

Breathing Organs: Has a cough—due to a cold—that has moved to the bronchial tubes. Has a loose discharge, particularly in the morning and in fresh air. Small drops of urine are expelled when coughing.

Digestion: An aversion to warm food and drinks; can't handle heavy, fatty meals, fruit, ice cream, cake, or eating too many different types of food at once. Food sits in the stomach like a stone. Rancid or burning, has bitter-tasting burps; nausea and vomiting of undigested food, diarrhea. Has a crampy and pressure-like stomachache after disappointments and being offended. Flatulence with colic-like pain, with loud noises from the stomach and intestine. Passes stool frequently; it varies in its consistency.

Urinary Tract: Painful, colic-like pressure on the bladder before urination; afterward, cramp-like pain, radiating into the thighs. Urge for more urination after just having urinated.

Female Genitalia: Menstruation too late, sparse, dark with clumps, and thick. No periods are ever alike. Delayed menstruation in young girls. Menopausal problems with frequent hot flashes and uterus prolapse.

Extremities/Back: Pain in the legs with restlessness and shivering. Pain in the limbs and rheumatic pain moves around quickly. Arms and legs fall asleep easily, W: the feeling of legs "hanging down."

Skin: Pale with tendency toward anemia. Rashes or small blisters (heat blisters) particularly on the neck, shoulders, arms, and legs; sometimes weeping. Tendency toward heat-related edemas in the legs. Skin breaks out when eating pork, especially in cases of late or sparse menstruation.

Fever: Constantly chilled, even in warm room, but can't handle heat. Not thirsty.

Sleep: Wide awake in the evening, and very tired in the afternoon. Has trouble falling asleep and wakes up before midnight. Often hands are crossed over the head or over the abdomen. One foot is placed outside the cover.

Worse: In the evening, for warmth in any form, for heavy, fatty foods, and lying on the left side.

Better: For fresh air, being outdoors, moving about, cold, cold food and drinks, attention, and sympathy.

PROVEN INDICATORS FOR PULSATILLA

Irritability, fear, phobias, insomnia, headaches, colds, hay fever, bronchial coughs, earaches, conjunctivitis, sties, stomach and intestinal problems, a feeling of fullness, flatulence, cystitis, a bad complexion, acne, rashes, heaviness in the legs, varicose veins, chicken pox, measles, mumps, and whooping cough.

RHUS TOXICODENDRON

Rhus toxicodendron is a proven remedy for skin rashes, colds, rheumatic complaints, and diseases of the connective tissue. Its key symptom is pain, a feeling as if something is being torn apart. All the complaints improve with motion.

CHARACTERISTIC SYMPTOMS

Mental/Emotional: Extremely restless, constantly in motion. Sad, indifferent, acts as if intoxicated. Restlessness during the night, must walk around.

Head: Has a heavy head. Face is swollen and red, with rash-like eczema that starts on the right side and moves to the left. Pain in the jaw joints; they make creaking sounds when the person chews.

Sensory Organs: Eyelids are red, swollen, and inflamed with ample yellow discharge; eyes are sensitive to light. Tongue has white coating with a red triangle at the tip; it is dry and rough.

Mouth: Fever blisters on the lips; the corners of the mouth are inflamed; the lips show a brown, dry crust.

Breathing Organs: Pain in the throat; swollen glands; mumps start on the left side. Hoarseness due to vocal stress. A dry, annoying cough after midnight, W: shivers, when an individual part of the body becomes cold. Stabbing chest pain with breathing difficulty.

Digestion: Bitter taste in the mouth; unquenchable thirst, particularly for milk. Slimy, foul-smelling stool. Diarrhea, pain along the thighs.

Extremities/Back: Pain in the tendons and ligaments. Limbs and back are stiff, as if paralyzed. Sciatic pain; lumbago. B: for lying on a hard surface and for motion.

Skin: Can't tolerate cold air. Skin is red, swollen, and itches severely. Has a rash with blisters. Chicken pox. Fever blisters.

Worse: During the night, when resting, lying on the back, lying on the right side, for damp/cold weather, and for getting soaked.

Better: For motion, warm, dry air, and rubbing.

PROVEN INDICATORS FOR RHUS TOXICODENDRON

Nervous restlessness, sensitivity to changes in the weather, headaches, rashes, colds, chicken pox, mumps, sprains, and pulled ligaments.

RUTA

Ruta is a indispensable remedy for injuries of the periosteum due to contusions, bruises, pulled tendons, pulled ligaments, and sprains. It is also a proven remedy for eye stain and is available in tincture form for external application.

SEPIA

Sepia is a far-reaching remedy for the treatment of general exhaustion, particularly that which is the result of years of being overtaxed on the job and/or by the family. It is a remedy that especially emphasizes treatment of the female organs, but it can be helpful for both men and women. Its central symptoms include weakness to the point of almost losing consciousness, being constantly cold, and pain that moves from the ground up. The complaints start primarily on the left side, and they all improve with movement.

CHARACTERISTIC SYMPTOMS

Mental/Emotional: Completely exhausted, burned out, feels abandoned, sad, dissatisfied, irritable, and moody. Has periods of anxiety. Sudden outbursts of rage and tears; sometimes verbally abusive. Very seldom talks about complaints, but cries when does so. Indifferent about family and job; works only because of a sense of responsibility. Avoids having people nearby.

Head: Unbearable headaches that come in waves at the beginning of menstruation. Stabbing headaches, also migraine headaches, from the inside out, particularly on the left side of the forehead, with nausea, vomiting, dizziness, and weakness. These symptoms cause the person to come close to losing consciousness. Sensitive hair roots; loss of hair. Pale yellow complexion, particularly around the mouth; dark circles under the eyes.

Sensory Organs: Vision problems, black spots "dancing" in front of the eyes, W: in the morning and evening. Skin rashes behind the ears. Yellowish "saddle-shaped" coloring over the nose. A thick, greenish discharge comes out of the nose; frequently there are crusts inside. A chronic cold, postnasal drip; must cough up clumps of mucus. The tongue is covered with a white coating but is clear during menstruation.

Teeth: Teeth ache from early evening until midnight.

Breathing Organs: A dry cough comes from deep inside the chest, as if the stomach was coming out, with a rotten-egg taste in the mouth. Tightness in the chest in the morning and evening. Breathing difficulty, W: sleep, B: quick movement. Has a cough due to an irritating tickle.

Digestion: Morning nausea, also during pregnancy, W: for the smell of food. Sometimes uncontrollably hungry; craves something sour. Has an aversion to fat. Can't tolerate milk. Sour-tasting burps, nausea, and vomiting after eating. A burning sensation in the pit of the stomach. Has stomach problems due to smoking. Everything tastes salty. Frequently constipated with a feeling as if there is a ball in the rectum, but can't push it out because if that is tried the pain shoots up. Incontinence, W: boiled milk.

Urinary Tract: Incontinence during initial stages of sleep. A chronically irritated bladder.

Male Genitalia: Cold, problems having erections, and loss of libido.

Female Genitalia: Menstruation is irregular, too late, and sparse or too early and too heavy; smells bad and causes a rash; often comes with headaches, migraines, and uterus cramps. Limp pelvic muscles with a sensation of a downward pull. Varied problems during menopause such as hot flashes, cold sweats, and uterus prolapse. A loss of libido with a strong aversion to sex.

Extremities: A weak back with radiating pain. Muscle twitches during the day and night. Legs are cold, tired, heavy, and feel "as if bruised."

Skin: Rashes with small bumps come after eating fish. Very painful corns, frequently inflamed. Varicose veins.

Sleep: Falls asleep late, wakes up often, and thinks somebody was calling. Sleepless in the early-morning hours, W: lying on the left side.

Worse: In the morning, at noon, in the evening, for cold, cold air, humidity, in warm rooms, after sweating, and before a thunderstorm.

Better: In a warm bed, for heat used therapeutically, motion, dancing, horseback riding, being outdoors, rest/quiet, and for sleep.

PROVEN INDICATORS FOR SEPIA

Irritability, sadness, depression, fear, sleep disturbances, tiredness, exhaustion, fatigue, a bad complexion, acne, rashes, corns, hair loss, cystitis, menstrual problems, morning sickness during pregnancy, and menopausal problems.

SILICEA

Silicea is a remedy with far-reaching effects in the treatment of general exhaustion, especially when it is a result of poor nutrition, and when it affects the skin and bones in particular. Its central symptoms include constantly being cold and chilly. All complaints improve through the application of warmth.

CHARACTERISTIC SYMPTOMS

Mental/Emotional: Paralyzing fear of failure and responsibilities. Easily discouraged, despondent, whiny, needful of protection, ability to think is blocked, W: mental stress, sensory stimulation. A phobic fear of needles.

Head: A dull, oppressive pain from the neck to the forehead; neuralgic pain in the face and teeth, W: changing to cold or damp/cold weather, B: for having head wrapped up keeping it warm. Scalp is constantly cold but sensitive, can tolerate only light, soft hats. Hair loss.

Sensory Organs: A sharp pain in the eyes; tear ducts swollen and highly sensitive to light. Has vision problems: letters run together. Sties. Ear noises. A dry cold with itching builds up only slowly; has a loss of smell and hard crusts inside the nose that bleed when coming loose. Colds easily include sinus infections, which cause oppressive headaches, then thick mucus discharge.

Mouth: Feels as if there is a hair on the tongue. Abscesses on the tip of the root of teeth. Gums are sensitive to cold air and cold water, and the edges of the lips are cracked.

Breathing Organs: A cold that involves the throat and chest and loosens up only with difficulty. A feeling of "needle pricks" in the tonsils; ear and salivary glands are swollen. A severe cough with a thick, yellow, lumpy discharge, W: lying down.

Digestion: Has a strong aversion against warm meals and meat. Asks for cold food and cold water. Can't tolerate alcohol. Swallows the wrong way easily, and food gets into the nasal passages. Has heartburn and stomach pain after eating; abdomen is hard, distended, feels cold inside. B: warm compresses. Always has to press hard when passing stool. Constipation before and during menstruation.

Female Breasts: Nipples are very sensitive, sore with deep cracks. When starting to nurse the baby, severe contraction of the uterus with slight bleeding.

Extremities/Back: A sensitive back, W: draft. Sciatic pain and cramps in the extremities.

Skin: Very strong-smelling head and foot perspiration, the rest of the body dry. Feet are ice-cold. Nails split easily, are very thick and deformed with vertical grooves, ridges, and many white spots. Abscesses. The formation of pus does not stop even if wound is open; pus is foul-smelling, thin, and the edges of the wound are inflamed and hard. Acne. Has a strong buildup of callused skin on the soles of the feet; dull, burning pain. Corns with dull, burning pain. Feet are ice-cold, with sharp, foul-smelling perspiration. *Silicea* is the main remedy for pulling out splinters of any kind, also from under nails. Pain in the navel.

Sleep: Falls asleep late, awakens before midnight and can't go back to sleep. Severe sweating of the head. Sleepwalking, W: new moon, and for lying on the side.

Worse: In the morning, for cold, draft, dampness, stress, when lying down, for lying on the left side, during menstruation, and in the winter.

Better: For warmth, covering the head, fresh air, and in the summer.

PROVEN INDICATORS FOR SILICEA

Fear, stage fright, phobia, shyness, insecurity, sleep disturbances, headaches caused by overwork, sensitivity to changes in the weather, colds, abscesses and boils, bad complexion and acne, calluses, brittle nails, hair loss, and injuries due to splinters.

STAPHYSAGRIA

Staphysagria is an important remedy for the treatment of injuries suffered from humiliation or insults. It has also proven very effective in supporting the healing of clean cuts.

CHARACTERISTIC SYMPTOMS

Mental/Emotional: Very dependent on the opinion of other people. Has severe attacks of rage after long-suppressed anger; is shaking with internal rage. Indignant. Has difficulty with assertion and suffers greatly because of it. Is numb, weak, and can't concentrate. Can't find sleep because of anger and worry.

Head: A dull, numbing pain in the forehead and back of the head; feels as if there is a ball stuck behind the forehead; the back of the head is numb. The scalp is sensitive with itching dandruff. The complexion is pale and sunken.

Sensory Organs: All senses are painfully overstimulated. Sties.

Teeth: The teeth ache, radiating into the ears, particularly during menstruation. Cavity-damaged teeth are black and crumbling. Bleeding gums.

Breathing Organs: Has a stabbing pain when swallowing, which radiates into the ears, particularly on the left side. Emotionally causes loss of voice.

Digestion: Colic-like pain after unpleasant events and worry. Ravenous appetite and hunger even after eating. Must have stimulants, including nicotine. Hot or blocked flatulence. Constipation.

Abdomen: Severe pain after abdominal surgery, also after cesarean section.

Urinary Tract: Irritated bladder, cystitis after birth. Burning in the urethra, even when not urinating. Feeling as if a drop is falling down. Pain after kidney stone operation.

Male Genitalia: Increased libido but erection problems.

Female Genitalia: Very sensitive; has irritated bladder after unfamiliar, intense sex.

Extremities/Back: Muscle and joint pain, feels "beat up." Back aches, W: in the morning before getting out of bed.

Skin: Especially good for clean cuts and tears and for dry, itching, and crusty rashes anywhere on the body.

Worse: For excitement, anger, indignation, worry, nicotine, and touch.

Better: For a night of rest, after breakfast, and for warmth.

PROVEN INDICATORS FOR STAPHYSAGRIA

Irritability, nervous headaches, sties, aching teeth, irritated bladder, cystitis, and cut and stab wounds.

SULFUR

Sulfur is a far-reaching remedy effective in loosening and preventing deep-seated blockages particularly relating to the skin. It works from the inside out. Its central symptoms are a strong aversion to water and standing as well as a distinct tendency for an illnesses to recur. All bodily orifices, like the nose, eyes, ears, rectum, are red.

CHARACTERISTIC SYMPTOMS

Mental-Emotional: Loves contact and being social, at the same time is often very self-important, ruthless. Has mood swings: is active, impatient, makes many plans, philosophizes, thinks of self as a genius; then again is depressed, irritable, without drive, lacks concentration, is forgetful. Wastes time lying about. Is sloppy, does not take care of appearance. Has a tendency to drink secretly.

Head: Pounding pain, also with dizziness, nausea, and vomiting, recurring periodically, W: for bending down. The scalp is dry and the part always hot. The scalp itches and burns after scratching. Hair loss, W: water.

Sensory Organs: The eyes are red during the day and itch during the night as if irritated by sand. The eyelids burn and are red and gummed up in the morning. Has a sensitivity to light. Nose entrance itches, burns, and is sore. The side of the nose is red with scales. For colds, also those that are chronic, with dry crusts, and a tendency for nosebleeds. The tongue is dry with a yellow-white coating; its tip and edges are red.

Mouth: The lips dry, bright red, and burning. Has a bitter, coppery taste in the mouth, particularly in the morning when waking up.

Breathing Organs: The throat is scratchy and dry with a sense as if there is a lump or splinter stuck in it. Hoarse coughing with shooting pain in the chest; head is hot, hands are cold. Has a dry cough, starting in the evening often with a burning, tightness in the chest, and breathing difficulty during the night.

Digestion: Nausea with dizziness and diarrhea in the morning. Gnawing sense of hunger around 11 A.M., but has had enough from just looking at the food. Sour burping with a taste of rotten eggs. Often intolerant of milk and baked goods. Noisy, watery, foul-smelling diarrhea in the morning. Sometimes alternates between diarrhea and constipation with a hard, ball-shaped stool. Hemorrhoids itch and burn. Rectum is sore and bright red.

Urinary Tract: Frequent urges to urinate, particularly during the night. Urine is hot and burning.

Genitalia: Itching, and the external portion is sore.

Extremities/Back: Often has a bent-over posture; does not like to stand at any time. Rheumatic back problems with pulling pain in the neck and shoulder area, particularly on the left side. Has drooping shoulders. The palms and soles of feet are hot and burning when covered up in bed, pushes feet out from under the cover. Deformed nails. Heavy legs and varicose veins.

Skin: Skin is red, dry, scaly, as if unwashed; every little injury festers. Severe itching and burning. Has rashes, pimples, cracks, and soreness.

Itching and burning, W: for scratching. All body openings are red. Has hot sweats of the head, hands, and feet. Hot flashes with outbreaks of perspiration lead to great exhaustion, underarm perspiration, W: menopause.

Sleep: Takes catnaps but awakens at the slightest sound. Can't go back to sleep after midnight until the early-morning hours.

Worse: In the morning, in the A.M., for washing, being in a warm bed, for alcohol, humid weather, rest, standing, and in the spring.

Better: Having many small meals, lying down, and in dry, warm weather.

PROVEN INDICATORS FOR SULFUR

Memory and concentration difficulties, sleeping disturbances, a bad complexion, acne, rashes, sore skin, nail biting, a feeling of fullness, flatulence, and menopausal problems with hot flashes and outbreaks of perspiration.

SYMPHYTUM

Symphytum is an important, supportive remedy for healing bruises, contusions (especially of the eye), and bone fractures. It is also available in tincture form for external application.

THUJA

Thuja is an effective remedy for problems of the skin and soft tissues. Its central symptoms are heavy perspiration with a sweet, garlic-like odor and a complexion that appears waxen, shiny or pale, often sunken. Problems usually occur on the left side. It is particularly effective for warts, diaper rash, and a bad complexion. *Thuja* is also helpful for tooth cavities at the gum line, periodontosis, and receding gums during menopause. Brittle nails and ingrown nails can also be effectively treated with *Thuja*. The tincture is also available for the external treatment of warts.

ZINCUM METALLICUM

Zincum metallicum is an important remedy for general weakness; it is also good for the treatment of anemia, particularly when this is due to years of stress, poor nutrition, and/or a severe, acute illness. Its key symptoms are slowed bodily function, constantly being cold, and trembling and nervousness with heightened and overly sensitive senses. All complaints improve when suppressed discharges (from the nose, through coughing, and in menstruation) are loosened up and, when suppressed, eczema breaks out.

CHARACTERISTIC SYMPTOMS

Mental/Emotional: Very weak, very nervous, irritated. All senses heightened and overly sensitive, sometimes—however—severely weakened, as if paralyzed or numbed. Lacks concentration, is forgetful. Sad, melancholy, uninvolved, does not care, tired, and has no drive.

Head: Pain in the back of the head, worst where the hair parts. Sometimes dizziness with the feeling of falling to the left side. The forehead is cool and the back of the head hot. The lips are pale and cracked at the corners.

Sensory Organs: All senses are heightened and overly sensitive, especially hearing; can't tolerate loud noise. Soreness and itching in the corners of the eyes. Blurred vision, particularly of one eye, especially prior to a migraine attack. Visual problems with great sensitivity to light after eye surgery, sees flashes of light and colored spots.

Breathing Organs: The throat is dry, as if choking; constantly tries to expel thick mucus. Has a bronchial cough with tightness in the chest and difficulty breathing, B: for discharging mucus.

Digestion: Ravenously hungry around 11 A.M. Eats greedily and fast, hickups afterward; has nausea, then vomiting with a bitter taste, and painful flatulence with a visibly distended and hard abdomen. Can't tolerate wine at all. Has heartburn and a burning stomachache after eating sweets. Constipation, producing small hard clumps. Particularly for children who have a watery, greenish-colored diarrhea.

Uninary Tract: Urination is only possible while sitting down and bending upper body back. Incontinence.

Female Genitalia: Menstruation is too late and heavier during the night; also fails to come on. Premenstrual complaints with nervousness, depression, muscle twitching, restless feet, and a painful spine; has pain in the left ovary. B: with the onset of menstruation.

Extremities/Back: Has a sensitive back and can't tolerate any kind of touch. Has a tired feeling in the shoulder and neck area, particularly after activities performed sitting down. Burning pain along the spine. Restless legs and feet, must constantly whip them back and forth, also during sleep. Nervous muscle twitching and lower leg cramps, a sense of numbness and spots that feel numb, especially in the lower legs, W: during pregnancy, after menstruation, and during menopause. B: during menstruation. Extremely large varicose veins.

231

Skin: A feeling of tingling and numbness. Itching in the back of the knees and thighs. A nervous rash. Eczema in case of anemia. Suppressed eczema, particularly due to external treatment with a salve. Frequent shivers.

Worse: in the late afternoon and early evening, for cold, touch, stress in any form, drinking wine, and before menstruation.

Better: While eating, during menstruation, for having discharge, and when expressing eczema.

PROVEN INDICATORS FOR ZINCUM METALLICUM

Nervous restlessness, menstrual and menopausal problems, restless legs, and varicose veins. IMPORTANT: *Zincum metallicum* does not go with *Nux vomica* and *Chamomilla*; do not use these remedies in succession. If the above-listed symptoms appear during the use of the zinc salve, discontinue its use; usually symptoms will disappear on their own.

TIPS ON CHOOSING A PHYSICIAN

Those who want to treat themselves and members of their family with homeopathic remedies should, no matter what the situation, look for a physician who is experienced in homeopathic treatment and has undergone homeopathic training. At the very least, try to find a reputable practitioner who has experience in homeopathy and is working closely with a physician. Avoid those who claim to heal every malady quickly.

Because of the growing interest in homeopathy among the general population, the sales of homeopathic remedies are also climbing. The result has been that some companies, often newcomers in the field, are bringing remedies on the market that in most cases consist of a combination of individual substances. These remedies are then offered to physicians and pediatric physicians, as well as to pharmacies for the population-at-large. All the above-mentioned professionals, while interested in natural healing methods, may have little or no experience in homeopathy. This can be a problem for two reasons: 1) Giving more than one substance at one time is warranted in only a very few cases. 2) Some of these combinations consist of several individual homeopathic substances that contradict each other in their characteristic symptoms. This fact is unknown to many physicians and pharmacists because they lack proper training in homeopathy. For that reason, if you want to use one of those combination remedies, always check with a physician or practitioner who is practicing classical homeopathy.

Of course, the best way to find a reputable and experienced homeopath is personal recommendation or word of mouth. Also, you can check with a pharmacy that carries an extended selection of homeopathic remedies; they will likely know a homeopath who practices in the area. Failing that, check the phone book listings under "Naturopathic Physicians" or "Physician—practicing homeopathy."

Indexes

HOMEOPATHIC REMEDIES

NOTE: **Bold** type indicates Materia Medica entry.

234

GENERAL

235

238

239